D0191523

AstroFit

The Astronaut Program for Anti-Aging

William J. Evans, Ph.D.,

Expert Adviser to NASA,

and Gerald Secor Couzens

Introduction by John Glenn

FREE PRESS
NEW YORK   LONDON   TORONTO   SYDNEY   SINGAPORE

FREE PRESS

A Division of Simon & Schuster, Inc.
1230 Avenue of the Americas
New York, NY 10020

Copyright © 2002 by William J. Evans and Gerald Secor Couzens
All rights reserved, .
including the right of reproduction
in whole or in part in any form.

Illustrations by Timothy J. Jeffs
Menus and recipes by Amanda Wells

FREE PRESS and colophon are trademarks
of Simon & Schuster, Inc.

For information regarding special discounts for bulk purchases,
please contact Simon & Schuster Special Sales at
1-800-456-6798 or business@simonandschuster.com

Designed by Karolina Harris

Manufactured in the United States of America

10 9 8 7 6 5 4 3 2 1

The Library of Congress has cataloged the hardcover edition as follows:
Evans, William J.
AstroFit / William J. Evans, Gerald Secor Couzens ; introduction by John Glenn.
p.   ill.   cm.
Includes index.
1. Aging—Prevention. 2. Longevity. 3. Aged—Health and hygiene. I. Couzens, Gerald Secor. II.
Title.
RA777.6.E94 2002
613—dc21   12660850

ISBN 0-7432-1681-4
       0-7432-1682-2 (Pbk)

To my children, Kelly, Christopher, Kate, Robert, and Julia, for putting up with my hours at work and time away (especially on weekends). It goes without saying that I would not have had the time to write this book without the remarkable support of my wife, Betsey. She always backs my endeavors with the greatest enthusiasm and love.

Acknowledgments

There are so many people I would like to thank for their assistance and support in helping me bring this book to you. My immediate gratitude goes to Senator John Glenn for the generous amount of time he spent discussing his own physical responses to space flight. His personal interest in the science of age reversal was and remains an inspiration to me. Thanks also to Mary Jane Veno, Senator Glenn's chief of staff, for her much appreciated assistance. Drs. Joan Vernikos and Victor Schneider at NASA have also provided considerable aid and support to our efforts.

Thanks in particular to Herb and Nancy Katz, friends and literary agents who guided me through the whole publishing process once again. Their faith in me, their unending support, and dedication to this project—along with a willingness to sharpen their blue pencils when necessary to improve the manuscript—has been extremely valuable and important. Without their keen direction, my research would not have found the widest audience possible.

Many thanks also to Fred Hills, my editor, for understanding the importance of this book, and for all the work he did to move it from manuscript to published book. Special thanks to Amanda Wells, who developed the meal plan and recipes that are so important to the AstroFit program. Thanks as well to Tim Jeffs, whose imaginative artwork adorns the pages. I am also grateful for the sage advice of Nellie Sabin, who carefully reviewed the manuscript from beginning to end and enhanced it immeasurably with her insights.

Gerald Secor Couzens worked closely with me on this project right from the start, helping commit my ideas to paper. In addition to speaking regularly on the telephone and e-mailing, he traveled to my lab in Little Rock to work out in my gym and speak with study participants to get a real sense of what AstroFit was all about. Thanks for helping make sense of my research and explaining it so eloquently for our readers.

A book like this makes extensive use of clinical studies. For every laboratory experiment discussed in this book, there was a group of dedicated subjects who regularly scheduled time for me and provided their effort, blood, and muscle tissue in the cause of science. I will be eternally grateful for their willingness to participate in our studies.

I would like to thank David Lipschitz, M.D., Ph.D., director of the Donald W. Reynolds Center on Aging at the University of Arkansas for Medical Sciences, for his continued trust and support. My colleagues at the Reynolds Center have been invaluable to me. Charles Lambert, Todd Trappe, Per Tesch, James Fluckey, Hannah Morse, and Nicholas Hays provide an atmosphere of intense curiosity, exploration, and hard work. Robert Wolfe at the University of Texas Medical Branch is a long-time collaborator and friend who has always provided generous time and support. David Costill at Ball State University, my mentor, demonstrated to me that life as a scientist could be not only intellectually challenging but also great fun.

—*William J. Evans*
Little Rock, Arkansas
May 2002

Contents

Introduction: A Talk with John Glenn

EVANS: Senator, you're such a splendid example of age reversal. You're vital. Strong. You move with grace. You exude health and vibrancy. I want to introduce the readers of my book to some of the lessons you and the NASA researchers learned from your nine-day *Discovery* voyage in 1998. In short, I want my readers to benefit from what we now know about the relationship between aging and space flight.

GLENN: That's what I was up there to do. To try and show the similarities between aging and space flight. To open the door, to start a process of finding what it is in the human body that turns these various systems on and off; comparing what happens to younger astronauts with what happens to older ones. Once we come up with more answers, we can have longer space flights than we currently are capable of right now. We couldn't do a Mars flight right now with what we know. However, as part of the process of preparing our astronauts to get to Mars, we will be able to take away the frailties we experience right here on Earth due to the aging process. That's why I was up there.

EVANS: And that was the inspiration for much of the research that led to this book.

GLENN: What you're talking about, Bill, is precisely the inspiration the public needs right now to understand the real meaning of age reversal. The aging process is natural, but getting weak and feeble is not. From my experience and your research, we know a long life of being strong, healthy, and never feeling that you're a day over forty is in the cards.

EVANS: That's what AstroFit is all about.

One

The AstroFit Promise

1

Reversing the Body's Aging, for Astronauts and for You

We ever long for visions of beauty,
We ever dream of unknown worlds.
—MAXIM GORKY

Astronauts will soon travel to Mars, a cold planet half the size of Earth, located more than 250 million miles away. No trip into space will have taken so long. No expedition will have involved such exhaustive, integrated preparation. As a society, we might react to the news of this incredible journey with awe and pride. Correctly, we would think of this adventure as the achievement of one of our greatest goals.

For me, however, there will be something more. For me, there will be a different kind of exhilaration, one that comes from the fulfillment of one's own goals. You see, the secondary benefit of the successful journey to Mars is the impact it will have on the struggle to reverse the aging process here on Earth.

The extensive plans for this three-year round-trip Martian voyage are well under way, and they entail the most comprehensive scientific preparation for any journey ever attempted. That is because prolonged space flight in microgravity—that's the word for almost zero gravity—results in remarkable physical changes within the body which are astonishingly similar to our journey into old age. *Traveling into old age is a damaging process we want to stop and reverse, especially as it concerns our muscles and bone.*

Weeks into their Martian adventure, the astronauts' muscle cells will atrophy. Some will be lost forever as these space travelers become as weak as most eighty-year-olds. Calcium will be leached from their bones at a greatly accelerated rate. Normal bone growth will be upset, leaving their bones pitted with craters and liable to fracture. Imagine the bones as being like a wool sweater that has been eaten by moths. The astronauts' balance will be extremely compromised. Their blood volume will be reduced, and their heart muscle will shrink. Their immune systems will be upset, and minor infections may pose major threats. Their bodies will be bombarded by radiation, greatly increasing the risk of cancer.

Turning Back the Clock

My job over the past few years has been to find effective ways to prevent the premature aging of the Mars-bound astronauts. As head of the Nutrition, Physical Fitness, and Rapid Rehabilitation Team of the National Space Biomedical Research Institution (NSBRI), I have been working on a program to prevent the astronauts from experiencing a physical deterioration equivalent to more than thirty years of aging on their journey to and from the Red Planet. The ultimate goal is to have a crew of astronauts land on Mars in great physical shape, with muscles and bones as strong and powerful as they were at liftoff nine months earlier—and to have them return to Earth in the same physical condition.

The good news is that a way to do this has been found. I can now share with you an age-reversal program that works for astronauts and will work for you. What I am proposing is revolutionary: a program that will allow all of us on Earth to take control of how quickly or slowly we age. The program is called AstroFit.

In my "Mars" laboratory at the Donald W. Reynolds Center on Aging at the University of Arkansas for Medical Sciences in Little Rock, I have been able to simulate a speeded-up aging process in order to see exactly what happens to muscle, bone, balance, and overall fitness. What normally takes place over the span of a lifetime, I can now observe happening in weeks, using as my test subjects healthy, active people in their twenties, thirties, and forties. My research has documented the advancement of aging, characterized by specific breakdowns and changes that occur in the human body in weightless conditions. In my lab, I am seeing what will happen to the astronauts on their journey to and from Mars.

As I became more involved in my NASA project, and the relationship between space aging and Earth aging became more apparent to me, I knew I needed to write this book. I wanted to share the AstroFit program with a wide audience so that it could have a significant and important impact on aging for all of us. Using special slow-motion muscle- and bone-building exercises I call E-Centrics, I can ensure that the Mars-bound astronauts will successfully withstand the serious health risks facing them. With special weight resistance training, they will learn how to protect their bodies from rapid aging.

By using a slightly modified version of the same program, you too can achieve age reversal, no matter what your age, no matter what your current physical condition. In this book you have the latest scientifically based information needed to forestall aging. Using the same research-based AstroFit program I have designed for the astronauts on the way to Mars, you, too, can achieve comparable protection and age reversal—no matter what your age. I've seen this happen firsthand so many times already, not only in my test subjects, but also in friends and family members who have followed the AstroFit plan for ninety days. Thanks to the innumerable breakthroughs that have come out of the NASA-sponsored research in my laboratory, and from other NASA labs around the country, we now have the means to stay younger and more vital for longer than at any other period in human existence.

Unhealthy Adaptations in Space

The Mars mission is now among NASA's top priorities, and a large contingent of dedicated NASA administrators and scientists around the globe is working to make this dream a reality within the decade.

I've had the privilege of working with many of them over the years while conducting my studies in human physiology. The ultimate goal of our collective research is to allow the crew of highly trained astronauts to switch on the afterburners of their spacecraft and gently ease it onto the dusty red surface of Mars. But how will a journey that will take three years—nine months going, eighteen months exploring the planet, and nine months returning home—and involve such exhaustive and integrated physical preparation of the astronauts be possible? More important, how will the astronauts, albeit highly trained and superbly conditioned, be able to survive the incredible physical rigors of this 500-million-mile roundtrip voyage?

I'm sure you've seen television clips of astronauts just back from outer space, unable to walk on their own after only a ten-day mission. For Mars-bound astronauts, the debilitation could be far worse. In traveling to Mars, these once healthy men and women could become old in every sense of the word—and at high risk of dying, either on Mars or later, after they arrive back home.

Muscle atrophy is a serious problem for astronauts in space and it progresses rapidly the longer they're aloft. On Earth, our muscles maintain some of their size and strength when we go about our daily chores, but they really begin to grow when we exercise them with weights. In the microgravity of space—which spacelings encounter within nine minutes of liftoff from Earth—the leg muscles soon become weakened from lack of use because astronauts "float" instead of walk and the leg muscles are no longer needed. The body senses that immediately and begins to rid itself of the muscle. To move in any direction, all the astronauts have to do is push with their arms against a fixed object, such as the wall of the spacecraft.

In this new environment, the large, powerful back muscles, which make up the most muscle tissue in the body, are suddenly free of all the load-bearing stresses experienced on Earth, and they, too, immediately begin to weaken. Although the skeletal muscles continue to control and move the body in space, the muscle fibers become significantly smaller in the absence of gravity. They also begin to alter, changing from slow-twitch fibers, which were once useful for support against gravity, to fast-twitch fibers, which are more useful for pushing. For every week an astronaut remains in space, his muscles typically shrink by 2 to 3 percent.

While weightlessness seems like everyone's dream of how to maneuver through life without much physical expenditure, it's actually a medical nightmare of gigantic proportions. Due to the extensive loss of muscle and bone that occurs, living in microgravity could turn the astronauts into old men and women decades before their time. Without taking proper countermeasures during the flight to Mars, they would arrive in an extremely weakened state. Stepping onto the Martian soil outfitted in their bulky space suits, they'd be so weak that even the most minor physical activity would seem difficult. They'd be too fatigued to turn the screwdriver needed to construct their prefabricated modular Martian dwelling. And with virtually no muscle power left, venturing out to explore and gather rock and mineral samples would be impossible.

Returning once again to the gravitational pull of Earth, the astronauts—once supremely conditioned forty- and fifty-year olds—would be transformed into the equivalent of slow-moving, infirm seventy- and eighty-year olds. Weak, dizzy, nauseated, and incapable of walking a straight line, their very survival would be jeopardized.

As an exercise scientist, I closely study people as they walk, run, swim, and lift heavy objects. I also examine them when they're sedentary and doing nothing more than clicking the TV remote control. Through my work on the Mars project, I've found that after an extended orbit of several weeks, astronauts suffer many of the same health problems that I see in our sedentary, aging population. They become weak, unstable on their feet, and extremely limited in what they can do. Ironically, what's happened to them is that their bodies have successfully adapted to life without gravity, only to find that these adaptations are quite harmful once back on Earth.

The human body is masterfully resilient. For thousands of years, it has withstood the rigors of famine, war, and natural disasters by adapting to its surroundings. When humans travel into space, their bodies similarly adapt to their new environment. But this elegant survival mechanism extracts a stiff penalty.

There is considerable evidence that most, if not all, of the "unde-

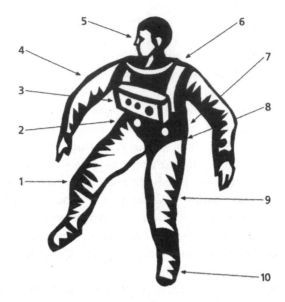

1. Legs: Calcium is leached from the bones, leaving them susceptible to breakage.
2. Stomach: Space sickness, a temporary condition, is caused by conflicting information that the brain receives from the eyes and inner ear.
3. Chest area: Blood pressure dips to a level appropriate for life in microgravity.
4. Arms: Muscles change from slow-twitch to fast-twitch fibers that are more useful for pushing.
5. Eyes: Eyes become the major source of balance information.
6. Heart: The heart muscle shrinks.
7. Lower back: Muscles atrophy.
8. Kidneys: Painful kidney stones may develop due to loss of calcium.
9. Legs: Floating causes leg muscles to deteriorate.
10. Feet: Feet no longer send balance signals.

sirable" changes in the body that occur in microgravity are necessary responses for the maintenance of body equilibrium. For example, the bodily fluids begin to redistribute almost immediately, causing blood pressure to dip to a level appropriate for the new environment but precariously low for life on Earth. While astronauts float through the cabin and perform breathtaking gymnastic feats, they aren't using their muscles and there is no impact whatsoever on their bones. In an environment where movement is effortless, bones begin to lose calcium and muscles shed unneeded mass. Space flight leaves astronauts too weakened to adapt to life on Mars or to function in Earth's 1-G force field.

The Mars Solution Becomes AstroFit

Protecting the astronauts as they change from earthlings into spacelings has been a formidable challenge, both for me and for other research scientists around the world. The mandate to return healthy astronauts to Earth from an extended Martian mission has forced us to try to fully understand how and why the body reacts to physical activity and just what happens when all physical force is removed from every aspect of daily living. Fortunately, our research has been yielding answers. From our body of work, I have derived a special program I call AstroFit that combines strength-training exercises with optimal nutrition. The AstroFit program will benefit astronauts in four vital ways:

Benefit 1. Their muscles will not shrivel. They will be able to
   maintain their overall strength and muscle endurance.
Benefit 2. Their aerobic performance will not decline. Their hearts
   will be able to sustain adequate blood pressure, and their aerobic
   capacity will be undiminished.
Benefit 3. Their bones will not become porous. Their skeletal
   systems will remain strong and intact.
Benefit 4. They will not age.

What's even more exciting to me is that you do not have to be an astronaut aboard a spaceship bound for Mars to experience these incredible benefits. In as little as ninety days, the AstroFit program will allow you to achieve the same age reversal as the astronauts.

Ninety Days to a New You

Performing the AstroFit program regularly comes closer to being a fountain of youth than anything modern medicine can offer. Although many people blame "getting old" on bad luck, fate, or poor genes, staying young is mainly a lifestyle decision that you make. In addition to making you feel thirty years younger, the AstroFit program will help you develop more strength than ever before. Your bones will become stronger, and you'll become steadier on your feet. In just ninety days, you will enhance your ability to compete in the workplace and on the sports field. Fatigue will be banished and your stamina will quadruple, giving you the energy to do the things you yearn to accomplish. You'll be able to live your life to the fullest. Live longer? Most likely. Live a fuller, more vital life? Most definitely.

There will be powerful psychological changes as well, starting with a huge boost in self-confidence. This belief in your skills and capabilities will be bolstered as you see yourself achieving your potential, getting stronger, and feeling more energetic.

You don't need a lot of equipment. You don't have to go on a wacky diet. There are no special pills or herbal concoctions. AstroFit is specifically designed to build lean body tissue—that's muscle—and to dramatically turn up your metabolism. When you speed up the process by which your body converts the calories in food to energy, you'll make steady and significant gains in how you look and feel, beginning with your first workout. In just ninety days, you will:

- *Go from fat to firm,* paring off pounds of excess body fat while still eating as much as you want of a fat-burning, muscle-nourishing diet. After just twelve weeks of dedicated exercise and proper nutrition, you will see a dramatic drop in your body fat composition and improvements in your muscle strength and firmness.
- *Put on pounds of fat-burning muscle.* Muscle is the most metabolically active tissue of the body. Think of muscle as an engine that is always turned on. Strengthening your muscles can help rev up your internal engine. After twelve weeks of E-Centrics, it will be like replacing your small four-cylinder engine with a

turbocharged V-8. Even when your muscles are at rest—for example, when you are sleeping—they keep burning calories. For every pound of muscle you put on with AstroFit, expect to burn an additional 100 calories per day. This will help reverse the slow but steady weight gain that is an all-too-common pattern among Americans.

- *Improve the functioning of your heart.* Like your other muscles, the heart becomes stronger and larger as a result of E-Centrics so it can pump more blood through the body with every beat. A fit heart will pump more blood at this maximum level and sustain the pumping longer with less strain.
- *Prevent or combat obesity and its cascade of dangerous health problems.* Most Americans eat not only too much but too much of the wrong foods—fast food, fried food, sweets, and "empty calories" with no nutritional value. To top it off, we're not physically active enough during the day. Therefore, it should come as no surprise that we've become a nation of fat people. Almost 35 percent of Americans are now considered obese. Obesity is a primary risk factor for heart disease and is linked to many other ailments as well, including diabetes, high cholesterol, high blood pressure, certain cancers, gallstones, and degenerative arthritis. Regular slow-motion E-Centric workouts, coupled with the sensible AstroFit eating plan, are the key to effective, permanent weight loss. Even small weight losses—10 to 15 percent of body fat—are associated with decreased cardiovascular risk, improved glucose tolerance, lower blood pressure, better cholesterol profile, and reduced symptoms of degenerative joint disease.
- *Bolster the production of insulinlike growth factor 1,* which directly stimulates muscle growth.
- *Build stronger, denser bones.* Strong muscles and strong bones go hand in hand. By targeting all the major muscle groups, the E-Centric program helps strengthen bones all over your body. The more weight you can lift, the more stress you can put on your bones—stress that stimulates more bone growth. More than 25 million Americans, many of them menopausal women, are thought to have osteoporosis, a disease of severe bone loss

that causes 1.5 million fractures a year, mostly of the back, hip, and wrist. About half of those who break their hips never regain full walking ability, and many of these fractures lead to fatal complications. By strengthening your muscles and bones and improving your balance, you reduce your risk of dangerous falls.

- *Prevent and reduce physical frailty.* It's now thought that by the time most Americans reach their seventies, more than one-fourth of the men and two-thirds of the women are unable to lift an object heavier than ten pounds, such as a bag of groceries, a laundry basket, or a small dog. Performing E-Centrics over the initial ninety-day training period will give you a guaranteed 5 percent boost in strength at every workout! No longer will you be daunted by any physical task, whether it be carrying luggage, opening jars, shoveling snow, or lifting your dog into the tub for a bath.

- *Improve your posture.* The E-Centric program works on building strong core muscles, particularly those of the abdomen (the *rectus abdominis,* the *external obliques,* the *internal obliques,* and the *transversus abdominis*). Posture is improved because strong abdominal muscles help support the spine and hold up your body throughout the day.

- *Improve your diet.* Part of the AstroFit program is nourishing your muscles with a protein-rich diet. Your muscles are fueled by calories from high-quality protein. If you don't consume a steady supply throughout the day, your body will "steal" protein from your muscles. The end result is that you will lose muscle. Also, without adequate protein, your body becomes less efficient at burning fat. My protein recommendation is *double* that of the current RDA. In order to ensure the steady utilization and release of energy, the protein-rich AstroFit food plan stresses the consumption of foods in the following percentages of total daily calories: carbohydrate, 60 percent; protein, 20 percent; and fat, 20 percent.

- *Combat excess blood sugar.* E-Centric exercises build muscle fast, increasing the sensitivity of cells to insulin, which, in turn, lowers blood sugar and the need for insulin. This helps prevent adult-onset diabetes. Lean muscle is the biggest "sponge" for soaking up glucose, the simple sugar that is the body's source of all energy. The less lean muscle you have, the greater your likelihood of developing excess blood sugar and diabetes. By adhering to the AstroFit program, you'll build lean muscle and help keep your blood sugar levels in the healthy range.

- *Improve your sense of balance.* Starting in their thirties, people begin to lose their balancing ability imperceptibly. This affects their daily living as well as exercise and sports routines. The AstroFit program will give you enhanced proprioception—a heightened sense of where your body is in space. Plus, when your muscles are strengthened, your balance improves and you become less injury-prone and less likely to fall. And when you do stumble, you will be able to right yourself more readily.

- *Reduce elevated levels of the stress hormone cortisol.* Stress is hard on the body; lowering stress levels can improve neural function and help prevent overall debilitation. When I work in my laboratory with the men and women in my studies, they are generally less tired, less angry, less tense, calmer, more focused, and happier. Your half hour of AstroFit training is "your" time, and the E-Centrics will help calm you, even if you are highly anxious. Exercise is great for your mental well-being because it gives you a beneficial "time out" from your worries.

- *Sleep like a baby.* You're guaranteed more restful, deeper sleep. E-Centrics help raise the core temperature of your central nervous system, lulling the body into a somnolence similar to that experienced after a warm bath.

- *Reduce depression.* The more you exercise, the more your body's cells increase their ability to use oxygen. Strong, muscular people are less likely to tire during the day, allowing them to work and play harder without missing a beat. Within two weeks of beginning AstroFit, you will feel an increase in energy and an enhanced mood. Even if you're not in good shape when you start, you can still achieve these wonderful benefits.

- *Boost your self-esteem.* You'll be surprised, but the psychological catharsis you undergo may match or surpass your physical changes. Performing E-Centrics regularly can improve your general feeling of well-being. Feeling healthier can raise your self-esteem, making you feel more confident, assertive, and attractive.

- *Enhance your sexual pleasure.* You couldn't ask for a better aphrodisiac. Not only does AstroFit improve your overall health, which then promotes better functioning of all of the body's systems, it also improves your body image. Because sex is a whole-body experience, it makes sense that you'll enjoy it more when your muscles, blood vessels, and nerves are performing at peak levels.
- *Reduce or eliminate joint aches and pains.* In a normal joint, each end of a bone is coated with cartilage, a tough, smooth, slippery cushion that protects the bones and reduces friction during movement. Osteoarthritis develops when cartilage breaks down or wears away, sometimes disappearing entirely, creating a painful bone-on-bone joint. Any joint may be affected, but the feet, knees, hips, and fingers are the most common. People with arthritis and osteoarthritis will greatly improve their condition and stay mobile and active by building muscle around the joints the AstroFit way. And remember, you can do this at any age.
- *Enhance your immune function.* Performing E-Centrics regularly will boost several key aspects of immune function. There's also evidence that people who exercise regularly have higher levels of InterLeukin 1 (IL-1), a natural substance that temporarily raises body temperature—producing fever—and helps kill invading organisms.
- *Improve your cholesterol levels.* Cholesterol, a waxy substance found in the bloodstream, helps form cell membranes, some hormones, and a variety of tissues. E-Centric training has the ability to boost protective HDL ("good" cholesterol) levels, while lowering LDL ("bad" cholesterol) blood levels. A high HDL level, defined as 60 mg/dl or more, is considered to be extremely protective against coronary artery disease.

AstroFit is revolutionary. Yet it's also basic, and, best of all, it works. Within these pages you will find everything you need to

My cholesterol was 240 mg/dl, and I hated the idea of having to take a medication to lower it, which is what my doctor wanted me to do. Instead, I made a pact with my physician: I would follow the AstroFit program for ninety days, and if I was able to trigger a significant drop in my cholesterol and a rise in my HDL levels, I wouldn't have to take the medication. My next cholesterol test showed that I was at 215 with an HDL of 50, a rise of 10 points. Dropping body fat, building muscle, and eating low-fat meals all played a role. I'm now convinced, and so is my doctor, that I will get my cholesterol below 200 and my HDL into the highest range.

—Roberta, age 34

revitalize and enhance your appearance, your health, and your life. This isn't a quick fix, but rather a rejuvenating lifestyle change involving special weight-training and balance exercises along with optimal nutrition for a high-energy, healthful way of life. The goal of AstroFit is to make you stronger, more active, slimmer, more mobile, more energetic, more vigorous, and more self-confident. In a word: youthful.

Why Slow-Motion E-Centrics?

One important aspect of my scientific investigation has been distinguishing what is true biological aging from what is a consequence of personal lifestyle choices. I'm convinced that much of the physical deterioration associated with the passage of time is far from inevitable, and that slow-motion E-Centric strength training to maintain and build muscle throughout life can reverse this decline.

From the studies of aging I have carried out with men and women as old as 100 years of age, what has become increasingly clear is that a sedentary lifestyle is a major aging accelerant. Lack of physical activity leads to a weakening of the body due to the loss of muscle, and also to an increase in the percentage of body fat. This is a slow, insidious process that can begin in our twenties and ultimately manifests itself in lower back pain, osteoarthritis, or a heart attack.

I've spent the better part of two decades uncovering the secrets of muscles, investigating how muscle fibers perform on a biochemical level and what type of weight training best stresses them and makes them get stronger. In the course of my research, I have developed the weight training program that is the foundation of my AstroFit program.

E-Centrics are very different from any type of weight training you may have done in the past. Even for an experienced weight lifter, the change in the raising and lowering cadence will take some getting used to.

Let me explain. Any weight-lifting maneuver, whether it's a biceps curl or a lunge, entails both a lifting phase and a lowering phase. The lifting phase is called the *concentric* phase. What is so novel—and extremely effective—about E-Centrics is that the focus is on the lowering phase of every weight-training exercise. This is the all-important *eccentric* phase of each exercise, the part that most people ignore when they lift weights.

Typically, what happens in weight lifting here on Earth is a struggle to bring up the weights and then—bam!—down go the weights, back to the starting position. The exerciser ends up missing out on what happens to be the most important part of the exercise. By lowering the weight *very slowly and smoothly,* you send the message to your brain that you need more muscle cells to help in the effort.

Muscles are made to contract. This is what happens in, for example, a biceps curl when you raise a dumbbell from your thigh, curling it up to your shoulder. However, when you perform an E-Centric biceps curl, you raise the weight in two seconds and then lower it slowly back down from your shoulder to your thigh in six seconds. First the biceps muscle contracts, and then it is powerfully stretched as you slowly lower the weight.

AstroFit is a safe, progressive strength-building program. The idea is to stress your body without straining it. At first, you perform exercises based on body-weight resistance, rather than dumbbells or gym weights. As you gain strength, you begin to add weights to your workouts. Each weight resistance E-Centric exercise is performed with a weight that can be lifted no more than ten consecutive times in perfect form. This means:

- Raising the weight in two seconds.
- Lowering the weight slowly in six seconds.

As you reach each strength plateau—where this type of lifting finally seems easy—you add 5 percent more weight at your next workout and introduce the muscles to the new resistance.

The body's response to this dual action is interesting: *within forty-
eight hours it builds significantly more muscle fiber than it would have
with a concentric-only maneuver.*

Ultimately, E-Centric exercises allow you to achieve the best results in the shortest time. In the process of exercising this way, the
muscle becomes stronger—*with 5 percent gains in strength achieved at
every training session for the first three months!*

It's Never Too Late

From the time that people first began studying humans in motion,
the prevailing belief was that as we aged we automatically became en-
feebled. The prevailing opinion was that those who remained strong
simply had better genes. "Survival of the fittest" determined who
would be self-sufficient and who would eventually need a cane, a
walker, a wheelchair, or a hospital bed. My groundbreaking research,
published in *The Journal of the American Medical Association* in 1990,
debunked that myth and just about every other previously held idea
regarding strength training and aging.

In a series of weight-training studies I conducted with sixty-, sev-
enty-, eighty-, and ninety-year-old men and women, strength gains
of up to 175 percent were observed in a matter of weeks, many participants increasing the size of their muscles by 15 percent with just
a few basic strength exercises. With those bigger, stronger muscles,
some of them were able to get out of their wheelchairs or put down
their crutches and canes, performing ordinary tasks that once had
been daunting and moving around unassisted as they had years before. Many of these people were surprised to find that the simple act
of building muscle with light—ten- and fifteen-pound—weights was
enough to transform their overall quality of life.

The only way to head off physical decline is with E-Centric resistance training, which gives us the power to continue to perform our daily activities right into our seventies, eighties, and beyond. Building new muscle keeps us active and vital. It's muscle that keeps us from becoming "old."

Jodie Gets Her Strength Back

Building upon my study findings, I've spent the past decade delving even further into the most efficient methods of maintaining and increasing muscle at any age. I've been able to take men and women and make their bodies, for all intents and purposes, years younger.

To determine how strong people are, I time them as they walk up a flight of stairs. Jodie, who was seventy-eight years old and had diabetes and hypertension, was out of breath almost immediately and didn't have the strength to go up the full flight of stairs. She shrugged her shoulders and said, "See. I told you: I'm old. Now you know what I mean."

I told Jodie not to give up. I had a surprise in store for her if only she would come back to my lab every Monday, Wednesday, and Friday for the next three months and perform seven simple E-Centric strength-training exercises. She agreed, and she never missed a training session in the next twelve weeks. After getting used to the special E-Centric movement on the weight machines, she dutifully raised and lowered the weights as I had instructed her.

On the ninetieth day, I took Jodie over to the stairs once again. She had completed thirty-six training sessions, and I wanted to show her how far she had progressed since her first workout. Taking out my stopwatch, I told her to go to the top of the stairs as fast as she could. Not only did she go up the full flight of stairs, but she went up as rapidly as someone thirty years younger.

Jodie had never thought it would be possible to regain the strength and vitality she had lost over the past decades. Happily, hers is not an isolated story. I see it all of the time with my test subjects of all ages who begin to lift weights. Think what Jodie's life would have been like if she had started this program in her twenties, thirties, forties, or even fifties!

Aerobic Exercise or Weight Training?

Although walking, biking, and swimming are all healthful aerobic activities that enhance the function of your heart and lungs, by far the best way to prevent or reverse muscle loss is through regular E-Centric strength-training sessions. Both types of exercise are good for you, but in different ways.

In a recent study, Danish investigators examined three groups of competitive athletes, all in their sixties and seventies. These test subjects trained and competed regularly as runners, swimmers, and weight lifters. As a control group, the investigators age-matched a group of sedentary older men and another group of active men who were twenty-four years of age, on average.

The remarkable finding of this study was that the men who had been swimming or running for most of their lives were no stronger than older men in the control group who were completely sedentary. These older endurance athletes certainly had much less body fat than their sedentary counterparts, but their muscle mass was just as minuscule as that of the sedentary seventy-year-olds. The older weight lifters, however, were much stronger than the older endurance athletes, and their muscle mass and strength were similar to that of the twenty-four-year-old men. Muscle biopsies revealed that the molecular structure of the muscles of the older weight lifters was similar to that of the young men. By contrast, the muscle composition of the swimmers and runners was similar to that of the inactive control group.

Aerobic exercise is definitely part of the AstroFit program. It's important to incorporate aerobic activity into your exercise week in order to maximize your cardiovascular fitness. However, the focus of this book is rebuilding muscle so you can maintain your strength and health for as long as possible. As you follow my AstroFit program over the next three months, you're guaranteed to add muscle no matter how old you are—effectively reversing the aging process.

If you already perform some type of aerobic exercise, you will be surprised to find that the strong muscles you get from AstroFit will enhance your ability to run, dance, cycle, and swim. In addition, your body's metabolic furnaces start to roar after each good weight-training workout. No aerobic exercise, no matter how great you feel afterward, will continue to burn calories once you're done.

The bottom line: You can run, bike, swim, or walk all that you want, which is great for cardiovascular fitness. But when it comes to building powerful, fat-burning, age-extending muscle, you have to lift weights E-Centrically to achieve the most benefit. Even regular weight training doesn't give the same results as AstroFit.

Women and E-Centric Training

E-Centric training is as important for women as it is for men. Unfortunately, the fear of developing oversized muscles like a male bodybuilder has kept many women away from weight training.

The development of muscle mass is a function of a woman's genetic inheritance as well as her training program. The circulating levels of testosterone—one of the primary hormones responsible for large gains in muscle tissue, as well as the development of the male secondary sex characteristics—are ten to thirty times greater in men than women. Therefore, it's extremely difficult for a woman to develop the size of muscles typically seen in men at comparable training levels.

My advice for women is to get rid of the notion that you will look like a bodybuilder once you start lifting weights. Women naturally have less bone and muscle than men, putting them at higher risk of osteoporosis and greater risk of disability as they age.

So what are you waiting for? If you want control over your body and spirit, a stronger, more powerful, self-confident woman is just a few E-Centric sessions away!

Suzanne Takes Her Fitness to the Next Level

A perfect example of a true believer is Suzanne, a test subject in one of my Mars studies. Suzanne ran three miles regularly and considered herself to be in excellent physical shape. At five feet, eight inches and 125 pounds she was thin, but the biggest muscles she had on her body were her hamstrings (located on the backs of the thighs). These helped power her along on her runs around Little Rock. Other than that, Suzanne had no significant musculature and barely any strength. When I tested her body fat percentage, it was 24 percent, which was too high for someone who put so much time into running.

A few weeks into the study, Suzanne realized she was nowhere near her true physical potential. Excited by the many positive changes she saw in herself—such as more energy, increased metabolism, and greater muscle definition—that came from her E-Centric workouts, she was not prepared to lose ground by going back to her aerobic-based workouts once the study ended.

In my laboratory, we have a special piece of equipment called the Space Yo Yo. It's a machine designed for E-Centric strength training in Earth's gravity or in microgravity. Suzanne had been training with the Yo Yo, but now needed a home workout using dumbbells that would provide the same muscle-building effectiveness.

I put together a program, and Suzanne bought a set of dumbbells. Over the next three months she trained E-Centrically three times a week. She started out with five-pound dumbbells, but she gradually moved up in poundage to keep pace with her tremendous strength gains. By the twelfth week, Suzanne was hoisting twenty-pound weights for some exercises and said that she'd never been so strong in her life. Her appetite had increased significantly, and she began consuming more low-fat, protein-based foods. Since she was developing metabolically active lean tissue, her body fat percentage started dropping to a more healthful level. As Suzanne's case illustrates so well, my AstroFit program enhances the whole person, producing a leaner, stronger, and more metabolically efficient body in the process. Most of Suzanne's clothing had to be taken in by a tailor, but this was a price she was happy to pay.

Fast, Tangible Results

With any type of aerobic exercise, you eventually make changes in how you look and feel, but you won't have much more muscular strength—plus it takes a while to realize any significant transformation. One of the interesting aspects of E-Centric training is that *half* of all the strength gains you make will come in the first three months, which means that you will be making significant increases in strength very quickly. This, of course, leads to immediate gratification and the motivation to continue the AstroFit program.

I've based the AstroFit program on three E-Centric workouts per week. Each one takes half an hour. This structure allows you to hit new benchmarks for strength, fat loss, and increases in muscle mass every four weeks. The program takes only three months or less to yield significant results. As an added bonus, it's extremely inexpensive.

In this book I provide you with my laboratory-based exercise and nutrition plan that's guaranteed to give you the means to slow or even reverse many of the most prominent aspects of aging. AstroFit works for the elite astronaut corps, and it will work even for sedentary people who have not seen the inside of a gym since their high school phys ed classes. Put in the time, and you'll reap the rewards quickly. At your very first workout, you will feel the changes in your muscles, and you'll see visible results six to nine workouts later.

2

The Science Behind AstroFit

That is the essence of science: Ask an impertinent question,
and you are on the way to a pertinent answer.
—JACOB BRONOWSKI

Shortly after John Glenn returned triumphant from space for a second time in 1998, I was invited by NASA and the American Federation for Aging Research to join him in an address to the National Press Club in Washington, D.C. Our topic that day was the similarities between extended space flight and aging.

The seventy-seven-year-old astronaut—the oldest by far of any of the four hundred people who had previously been in space—had just completed a successful mission aboard the space shuttle *Discovery*. In addition to monitoring Glenn's sense of balance during the 144 orbits of Earth, fellow crew members collected data during the mission to study the rate at which his muscles absorbed protein in microgravity.

Glenn was certainly not new to space travel. Thirty-six years earlier, as a member of the pioneering seven-man Project Mercury program, he had rocketed into the history books as the first American to orbit the earth. His 1962 solo voyage had lasted a little less than five hours as he circled the globe three times. Enthralled by the adventure, Glenn had always wanted to go back, but other things had gotten in the way, not the least of which had been his distinguished career in the U.S. Senate.

Upon hearing of the upcoming seven-person *Discovery* trip and having become free of his legislative obligations, Glenn immediately began lobbying NASA to get a seat on the shuttle. His stated goal was the unique opportunity to study the science of aging. It was an offer that made sense on many levels.

As I explained to the journalists, Glenn's Project Mercury team of astronauts was perhaps the most thoroughly studied in human history. Each had exhaustive medical records that had started in the 1950s and had been continually updated and maintained to the present. Glenn had felt that physical changes in an older astronaut could provide a vast amount of valuable information that might help shed some light on the aging process.

Glenn had always had a strong interest in aging issues. In his twenty-four years in the Senate, he had been a champion of the elderly, as well as something of a lay scholar on the biology of aging. It had not escaped his notice that some of the changes the body goes through as it ages—the breakdown of muscle and bone, for example—are identical to the changes the body goes through in microgravity. What better way to study both phenomena than for NASA to send a senior citizen into space?

If John Glenn's extraordinary trip did nothing else, it blasted away the mistaken notion that all elderly people are frail and weak. Glenn, the world's oldest astronaut, handled the rigors of weightlessness as well as astronauts younger than half his age. Postflight analysis by my colleague Dr. Arny Ferrando showed that Glenn had suffered no more loss of bone mass or muscle than the other astronauts on the flight with him. And his heart rate before, during, and after the trip was actually slightly better than many of the younger male astronauts.

Glenn had "the right stuff" in older age because he had taken good care of himself throughout his life. John Glenn's take-home message for the National Press Club audience, and for all of us, is that there is no magic pill you can take that will make you live forever. However, strength training, regular aerobic exercise, and good nutrition offer the best chance for living a long and productive life until your eighties and beyond.

The Space Yo Yo

One spring morning, I stood by in my lab as Dr. Per Tesch, notebook in hand, quickly adjusted the large plastic wheel on the Space Yo Yo. In the world of muscle and strength experts, Per Tesch is king. The forty-eight-year-old professor of physiology at the Karolinska Institute in Stockholm, Sweden, has been working with me in my lab for more than a year and is scheduled to continue with my Mars project for the next few years.

Not only a brilliant physiologist, Tesch is also an impressive physical presence. A flat-water kayaker on the Swedish national team, six feet one and 185 pounds, he is lean and muscular and moves about my lab with the litheness and grace of a large cat. And he knows about muscles, not only from his own personal rigorous workouts but from his years of research on skeletal muscle adaptations to weight lifting. He has published more than 150 studies on muscle. His more recent breakthrough studies using magnetic resonance imaging (MRI) on muscles have helped uncover the best ways to build and sculpt lean muscle tissue.

The Space Yo Yo is his ingenious black iron and chrome invention we had been testing on a series of volunteers for the past several months. This brilliant Swedish scientist, a world-renowned expert on muscle growth, scribbled some more numbers in his book. If all goes according to plan, Tesch's special patented weight-training creation will become the primary exercise tool in the Mars space capsule.

The beauty of the machine is that it will allow astronauts to train their muscles effectively on the way to Mars without using traditional iron weights. This exercise device, which looks quite similar to an exercise machine you'd see at your local health club, is actually like nothing ever before invented.

To use a traditional leg-strengthening machine, you must sit down on the edge and place your lower shin under a thick roller pad that's attached by a cable and pulley to a stack of iron weights. By forcefully raising your leg up to parallel, you stress your quadriceps muscles against the weight. On Earth, it's the heavy iron weights

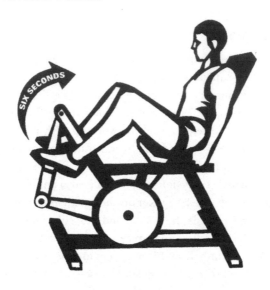

The E-Centric Workout involves two phases, a concentric phase (two seconds up against gravity) and an E-Centric phase (six seconds down against gravity). In this exercise, the E-Centric phase occurs while resisting the machine as it pushes the legs up.

that provide the resistance, making it extremely difficult to raise and lower.

In the weightlessness of space, iron weights are useless exercise tools, since even the weakest person could easily lift something weighing thousands of pounds. The beauty of Tesch's exercise device is that it provides tremendous resistance—and significant muscle-building capability—without any weights.

On the Yo Yo, the exerciser simply adjusts his lower shin against the resistance pad and then raises his leg. When he does so, a two-inch-wide length of nylon strapping attached to the pad provides a high level of resistance as it is pulled out from an axle that's connected to a large plastic flywheel. This, says Tesch, is the heart of the Yo Yo. The flywheel, about the size of a thirty-gallon garbage pail top, sits near the base of the machine at the back. As the nylon strapping plays out, the flywheel starts turning rapidly, just like a child's Yo Yo.

Once the leg is almost at parallel, there is suddenly a strong reverse pull on the leg pad. This means that the Yo Yo has reached the end of its tether, and, just like the toy spinning rapidly at the end of its string, it begins to pull the nylon strapping back, wrapping it quickly onto its axle.

Lifting the leg up against the resistance provides the *concentric* muscle contraction. Resisting the strong tug of the Yo Yo as it pulls the leg back to the starting position is the more powerful *E-Centric* muscular contraction—and this is how muscle is strengthened to its maximum.

Erica's Yo Yo Workout

Erica Gordon, a forty-one-year-old test volunteer decked out in a white T-shirt, lycra shorts, and running shoes, was sitting patiently on the Yo Yo, ready to perform a knee extension exercise that would strengthen her upper leg. She adjusted her right shin under the pad and then gripped the handles at the side of the machine. She was ready to exercise again. Tesch clicked his stopwatch and told her to begin. She slowly kicked her leg up and then straight out, which she did with some ease. Tesch clicked his stopwatch again and quickly noted the time in his book. Two seconds. This was the concentric contraction of the leg extension exercise, the first movement of the dual lifting and descending phase.

Gordon's quadriceps muscle, just above her knee, was well developed from her daily ten-mile bike rides, and it was obvious that she was strong and fit. Once her leg was completely horizontal to the ground, there was a slight whirring sound. The Yo Yo flywheel began to reverse, and the strapping suddenly began to pull the pad—and Gordon's leg—back down toward the machine.

The E-Centric phase, the second half of a strength-training movement—that is, the lowering phase—was beginning. To be effective at muscle building, this E-Centric portion should take *at least three times as long* as the concentric phase of the exercise. That's because Tesch's research has proven over and over that it's in the E-Centric portion that the most muscle growth takes place.

E-Centrics are the fastest and most effective way to strengthen muscles for one simple reason: because of the great stress placed on the muscles, microscopic tears develop in the muscles being exercised E-Centrically, and this provides a powerful stimulus for them to "wake up," rebuild, and grow so that they become stronger than before. Muscle growth happens primarily because the muscle cells under the E-Centric stress produce a substance called insulinlike growth factor 1 (IGF-1), which directly stimulates muscle growth. As a result, the muscles become stronger and *hypertrophic,* or larger.

Tesch became animated, and, like an agitated NBA coach roaming the sidelines during the final seconds of a close playoff game, he shouted encouragement to Gordon: "Resist the pull! Come on, you can fight it, Erica. Now, again. Two up, six down!"

The intensity of the session was visible on Tesch's face. He wanted Gordon to get a maximal workout, and he had to encourage her to work harder. She continued, gritting her teeth as she pushed up and then resisted the Yo Yo as it pulled her leg back down.

This morning, Tesch had already taken Gordon through five other exercises on the Yo Yo. Two exercises were specifically designed for her midsection, one for her arms, one for her shoulders, and another for her lower back. Although Gordon was new to E-Centrics, she quickly grasped the core concept of the E-Centric program: *Raise the body part in two seconds, then lower it against the resistance, taking six seconds to get back to the starting point.*

Beads of sweat quickly formed on Gordon's brow as she continued with the leg exercise. Her quads had turned pink as blood flooded the working muscle, which now stood out in stark relief on her leg. With Tesch encouraging her to fight the Yo Yo, she kicked up and then resisted as best she could through ten nonstop up-and-down repetitions. Within ninety seconds or so it was all over; her foot was flat on the floor, and she was breathing heavily.

"Yes, you did it. Wonderful. You did great!" said Tesch, giving an enthusiastic thumbs up.

Gordon shook her head slowly. "Nothing like it," she said. "It felt like my thighs were literally on fire."

She quickly toweled off. I handed her a container filled with

"AstroBlast," and she took a deep gulp. This was the protein-rich concoction of amino acids we were testing as a muscle replacement and growth "fuel" to be taken by the astronauts after each E-Centric workout en route to Mars.

Next on Gordon's schedule was an appointment at the university hospital next door to have an MRI scan taken of her leg, arm, abdominal, and back muscles. These imaging tests would ultimately determine what precise effects the Yo Yo's E-Centric forces had had on her muscle growth.

Since we had already done many of these imaging tests in the past few months, Per and I already knew that the results would be awesome.

My Body-Wasting Studies

The wasting of the body's muscles and bones in space is similar to what we see over time in people on Earth who don't exercise. The parallel is so close that to simulate the effects of space flight, we find volunteer test subjects and physically immobilize their muscles in what we call body-wasting studies.

One way to mimic the various negative physical effects of extended space flight on the body's muscle is to have a test subject wear one shoe with a specially fitted sole that is built up five inches. As the person uses a pair of crutches to get around, this raised shoe keeps the other foot from ever touching the ground. In physiology circles, we call this a unilateral leg suspension. The beauty of it is that it eventually causes the muscles of the suspended leg to wither over a period of three to five weeks. These tests are relatively inexpensive to carry out but sometimes problematic because the test subjects cannot always be monitored.

The second way to test the volunteer subjects is more costly and complicated: a group of men and women is assembled, and they are sequestered in a facility and confined to bed for a month, creating complete physical inactivity, which causes bone demineralization and atrophy of all of the muscles of the body.

For the Mars project, I had to perform both types of in-depth body-wasting studies. Ultimately, the research was extremely valuable because it let me see just how effective my E-Centric exercises were in keeping muscles from shrinking.

I told the volunteers in the two studies that they would be participating in a very important dress rehearsal for the astronauts in space. What we would find out from the host of muscle and skeletal changes that were taking place in them would ultimately be used to ensure the safe passage of the astronauts to Mars and back.

The Leg Suspension Study

I gathered twenty test subjects in my lab and explained to them that for the next five weeks they would have to wear their special elevated shoe every day. Among the group were a high school basketball referee, several graduate students, some homemakers, and some salespeople, who would continue their normal activities as best they could during the course of the study.

I made it clear that they were to put the shoe on in bed before they got up in the morning and wear it everywhere they went throughout the day, including into the shower. Their left foot was never to touch the ground. Ever. There were to be no exceptions.

Daily check-ins at the lab were mandatory to ensure that this order was being strictly followed. Violators would be eliminated from the study. Jay Trieschmann, my program coordinator, would be sent out to follow anyone we suspected of cheating, which in this case

---

Getting around on one leg was difficult, but I managed. However, what I found to be the most surprising was how much my left leg actually shrank in size during the weeks I was using crutches. This ultimately made me realize how important it was for me to be active and move my body as I got older.

—*Jack, age 44*

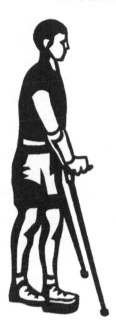

meant walking on two feet. Surprise visits would be made at their places of work and also at home, and leg temperatures would be taken.

By putting a thermometer against their calf muscle, Jay would be able to tell if they were complying with the study protocols. Within twenty minutes of not using the calf muscle, the muscle temperature drops anywhere from three to five degrees Fahrenheit. If Jay detected a high reading, it meant that the leg had been used for walking; blood was pumping into the calf muscle of the leg, causing the temperature to go up. In addition, we would also regularly measure the circumference of the muscle to make sure that there was the expected amount of stasis, or shrinkage, consistent with lack of use.

During the study, ten volunteers were randomly selected to exercise their suspended left leg on the Space Yo Yo three times a week. Each performed four sets of seven repetitions of the leg extension exercise at maximal effort. The total exercise time was about ten minutes per workout. The other ten test subjects would come to the lab daily for checkups, but they weren't allowed to exercise.

Before everyone was sent off on crutches, a biopsy was taken of each calf muscle; a small piece of muscle tissue was extracted that would be examined under a microscope to note the muscle cell size. An MRI of each leg muscle was also performed to give us precise measurements of muscle size and create additional baseline data. In five weeks, these tests would be performed again and the results compared to determine the outcome.

The study went according to plan, with only one volunteer asking to leave. The men and women who used the Yo Yo were conscientious and worked hard on the machine following my instructions: slowly and in control; two seconds up, six seconds down.

After the second week, I could tell the Yo Yo was working just by looking at the left leg muscles of the test subjects. I could see that they appeared strong, even after fourteen days of not being used. By contrast, it was plain to see that the nonexercisers' leg muscles had become flaccid and were visibly shrinking in size. Our final muscle biopsy and MRI tests gave me the ultimate answers I needed:

- Our nonexercising volunteers showed a *significant decrease* of 10 percent in lean muscle mass over the five-week period. At the end of the study, most had difficulty walking on two feet and had to participate in an extensive rehabilitation program at the Reynolds Center to restore their muscle size and strength.
- Our Space Yo Yo exercise group did more than maintain their muscle size. In fact, they showed a *significant increase* of 9 percent in muscle mass with this relatively limited amount of weekly E-Centric exercise.

This was the first time that I had ever done any type of resistance training in my life, although both my husband and daughter work out with weights regularly. After the study, I continued with my E-Centric training on my own and have shown Rick and Susan how to perform the two seconds up, six seconds down workouts.

—Connie, age 40

The Bed-Rest Study

The special lab across the street from my office at the Reynolds Center has private rooms, each outfitted with two beds, night tables and lamps, telephones, computers with Internet hookup, and small washbasins, plus a television and VCR. Each room is sterile, quiet, and efficient.

It is here that I will soon sequester sixteen male and female test subjects who volunteer to be in my Mars bed-rest studies. NASA may also be sending female astronauts to Mars, which is why this bed-rest study will include women. Everyone's charge: *never* get out of bed for four weeks. For bathing, there will be special horizontal showers that go over the bed. Daily toilet needs will be accomplished within the confines of the beds with bedpans and urinals.

Once the subjects take to their beds, they will be like the astronauts who will eventually lift off from Cape Canaveral on the Mars journey. One week of complete bed rest will be the equivalent of more than one year of aging on their skeleton.

And there they will stay for days on end, reading, eating, chatting, watching television, and sleeping. Strict limitations will be placed on all their movements in order to best atrophy all their muscles. This is the only way to mimic the muscle and bone loss that will occur when the astronauts are floating within their space capsule.

Four days a week, nine of the volunteers will work on strengthening their upper-, middle-, and lower-body muscles on a specially modified Space Yo Yo that will be wheeled into their rooms. The test subjects will move over from their beds to the exercise machine, their feet never touching the floor. For the next thirty minutes they will perform a series of E-Centrics under the watchful eyes of my lab assistants. After performing three sets of eight repetitions of leg extensions, knee flexions, "lat" pull-downs, and chest presses—two seconds up, six seconds down—they will be finished for the day and go back to their sedentary ways.

The E-Centrics will provide a nice break in the subjects' otherwise quiet days, but, more important, it will give me the vital information I need to see what strength-training exercises can do to prevent mus-

Similarities Between Space Flight / Bed Rest and Aging

	SPACE FLIGHT/BED REST	AGING
Muscle mass	Decreased	Decreased
Bone density	Decreased	Decreased
Aerobic capacity	Decreased	Decreased
Strength	Decreased	Decreased
Balance	Decreased	Decreased
Sleep	Decreased	Decreased
Insulin sensitivity	Decreased	Decreased
Growth hormone	Decreased	Decreased
Cortisol production	Increased	Increased
Risk of cancer	Increased	Increased

A great many of the changes we had previously thought to be caused by aging are either directly caused by physical inactivity or else exaggerated by it. These ten examples are important biomarkers for advancing age that can be changed, modified, or reversed with regular E-Centric training.

cles from shrinking. Based on several preliminary studies that I and my colleagues in the metabolism group at the University of Texas at Galveston have already carried out, over the twenty-eight-day study period, I expect our nonexercising men and women volunteers to show a *decrease* in overall muscle strength and a *decrease* in overall muscle size. Our exercising men and women volunteers will show a *30 percent increase* in overall muscle strength and a *5 percent increase* in overall muscle size. Our nonexercising men and women volunteers will show *increased losses* of body protein stores, a drop in glucose tolerance and insulin action, and a loss of bone density. Our exercising men and women volunteers should show *minimal losses* in nitrogen, which is a sign that they are able to maintain critical protein levels. The E-Centric exercises will *significantly increase* the rate of skeletal muscle protein synthesis, helping the muscles to grow.

What will be made very clear by this study is that bed rest results in a rapid and extreme loss of muscle mass. The muscles that are af-

I never exercise and was pretty weak physically before the study began. I was put in the nonexercising group, and after a month, what little strength I had in my leg was totally gone. I felt so old!

—Abby, age 36

fected first will be the postural muscles, the muscles that keep us standing up all day long. However, all muscles are eventually negatively affected as the bed rest continues. In addition, the oxidative capacity of the muscles is diminished—that is, the muscles lose the ability to utilize oxygen during physical activity. To make matters worse, the number of capillaries going to the muscles decreases, limiting their capacity to deliver oxygen directly to muscle cells. And the mitochondria, the "powerhouses" of the muscle cells, decrease in size, further limiting the ability of the muscles to work.

Perform E-Centrics, and this won't happen to you. My research clearly shows that the rapid losses of muscle and bone can be prevented, with significant gains made in reversing the processes if they have already begun.

Slow-Motion E-Centrics Are the Centerpiece of the Personal Home Program

Important controlled studies like the ones I've performed in my lab further solidify the connections among E-Centrics, muscle growth, and muscle and bone preservation. The scientific information is indisputable: E-Centrics offer a sound and comprehensive training regimen for our astronauts on the way to Mars—*and* for everyone here on Earth.

The volunteers who used the Space Yo Yo in my studies found that they finally had an exercise routine that worked. Not only did they become stronger and better toned, but the E-Centric workout was a routine that they could easily complete.

Many of the volunteers were looking forward to continuing the

I thought I had enough muscle and strength and that building more would be something only bodybuilders did. The Yo Yo workouts highlighted my weaknesses, helped me develop more strength, and contributed to an overall sense of well-being that I never had before.

—*Vernon, age 37*

E-Centric exercise in the future. With the study coming to an end, and since they would no longer have access to the Space Yo Yo, they wanted to know how they could perform the E-Centrics at home or at their health club.

I discussed their concerns with my colleagues at the Reynolds Center, as well as with some experts from the Nutrition, Physical Fitness, and Rapid Rehabilitation Team of the National Space Biomedical Research Institution (NSBRI). What became clear to me was the need for a comprehensive home program that would pull together all of the essential pieces we were using with the astronauts. I wanted to combine my new findings about E-Centrics with the latest information on balance, osteoporosis, and nutrition. The aim was to develop a practical home program that would become the foundation for a long, healthy, vibrant life. That is how the AstroFit program was developed.

My Life Extension Prescription

The goal of AstroFit is straightforward: regardless of how old you are, how much you weigh, how strong you are, and your current physical status, follow the program for three months and you will create a dynamic lifestyle of exercise and nutrition that will reverse your aging process. AstroFit is graduated and takes all levels of health and fitness into account—you progress according to *your* individual ability. You will be lifting a weight that is right for you and your strength. Whether you have trained your whole life or are coming back to the exercise lifestyle after a lengthy absence, AstroFit is designed to provide you with the means to stay healthier for a lifetime.

A Lesson from Bears

Imagine that you volunteer to participate in one of my bed-rest studies. However, instead of twenty-eight days, you have to stay in bed for six months! You've already read what twenty-eight days of bed rest does to muscles and bones. Longer periods are even more damaging. It's now estimated that staying in bed for 180 days will cause you to lose as much as 90 percent of your muscular strength.

If that's so, then why don't black bears—which hibernate for as long as seven months out of the year—lose all of their muscle power during their long sleeps? Instead, they emerge from their winter hibernation with about 75 percent of their former strength.

Researchers from the University of Wyoming recently studied six sleeping bears by connecting special equipment to the muscle that bends the bears' rear foot up and down. Based on the results, the scientists have theorized that shivering, a natural way to give the muscles a workout by causing them to exert force against one another, could be just enough of a workout to keep the bears' muscles strong. Uncovering the secret of how bears maintain muscle strength may one day help our astronauts better cope with the lengthy confinement of long-term space travel.

The choice to live better and longer is yours to make. With AstroFit, I'm offering you the longevity prescription. Now it's up to you to fill it. Take charge of your life. Make the commitment now to building muscle and bone, eating right, and injecting doses of vitality into your life each and every day.

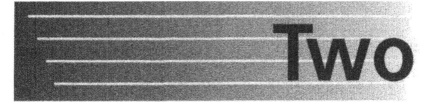

Two

Preparing for Transformation

3

Building Muscle

Aging seems to be the only available way to live a long time.
—DANIEL-FRANÇOIS-ESPRIT AUBER

For many years, exercise physiologists and most physicians strongly recommended aerobic exercise as being the best and only type of exercise that improved health. It is clear that regular aerobic exercise—running, swimming, bicycling, dancing—does prevent a host of chronic diseases and helps boost longevity. But what about lifting weights and moving the muscles against resistance? Where did that fit in? Not long ago many exercise experts thought that weight lifting was for "muscleheads," bodybuilders who spent hours every day hoisting weights without accruing any positive health benefits.

How wrong most experts turned out to be.

When I became the director of the Human Physiology Laboratory at the Tufts University Human Nutrition Research Center on Aging, I began examining the health and fitness of older people. The one common feature that every test subject exhibited, whether seventy, eighty, or one hundred years old, was extreme muscle weakness and a significant loss of muscle mass.

So what was the "cure"? It turned out to be resistance exercise, something the serious muscleheads already knew. I became convinced that the only way we could reduce the symptoms of a lifetime of inactivity was to have our older subjects lift weights several times a week. As I've already mentioned, the results of these studies were nothing short of spectacular. Strength training created strong ligaments and tendons, which supported the joints, improved balance and flexibility, and decreased the likelihood of falls. Bone density increased as well, helping stave off osteoporosis. I also noticed that regular weight training bolstered the subjects' self-confidence. As their strength increased, so did their energy levels, and with that came spontaneous bursts of physical activity throughout the day.

However well my frail, elderly test subjects responded to the resistance exercise programs, it became clear to me that the best way to combat the age-associated loss of strength and muscle mass was to prevent it from occurring in the first place. I was confident that if intervention began much earlier—if people began lifting weights several times a week starting in the teen years—we wouldn't be seeing such great numbers of frail elderly people.

NASA soon got this weight-training message as well. The exercise program recommended for astronauts in space had been walking or running while tethered to a treadmill by bungee cords, but NASA came to understand that the most effective way to counter the loss of muscle, strength, and bone in space is with E-Centric strength-training workouts.

We Are All Very Muscular

The audience was incredulous. The men with the potbellies and the women with the ample hips simply didn't believe me.

"You're all extremely muscular," I told them again, looking out over the crowded auditorium in Little Rock one unseasonably chilly spring evening. Many who had come to hear my talk about strength training and aging were surprised. They knew that they didn't look anything like the prototypical athlete, which is what most people think being muscular really means. Some thought they were out of shape. Others came right out and said that they were just too heavy. To a person, though, they all admitted that they felt older than they should. What my audience didn't realize was that each one of them had the *potential* to burn off excess body fat and to develop the wide array of skeletal muscle that's hiding just beneath the surface of the skin.

The Three Types of Muscle

Our muscles help us do everything throughout the day. From the beating of our heart, to the blinking of an eye, to lifting groceries, to digesting food, our muscles are at work. As much as 45 percent of a man's body by weight and up to 35 percent of a woman's body by weight is muscle. Each muscle consists of 75 percent water, 20 percent protein, and 5 percent salts and fats. The beauty of muscle is that with the help of regular E-Centrics you can rebuild the strong muscles of youth, giving you more muscle mass than you ever had before.

Your body contains 650 muscles, of which about 620 are called *skeletal* muscles because they are fastened to the bones of your skeleton by strong, rope-like lengths of connective tissue called tendons. These are the muscles that we can see and feel. The main function of the skeletal muscle system is the movement of the body's bones to provide power and strength. These muscles are also called *voluntary* muscles because you can contract them—tighten them up—at will. With the E-Centric training program, you will be developing the major skeletal muscles of your upper, middle, and lower body. These muscles produce more heat, consume more calories, and receive more blood flow than any of the body's other muscles.

Skeletal muscles come in pairs. The *agonist* muscle moves a bone in one direction, and the *antagonist* muscle moves it back the other way. Take a look at your biceps on the front of your upper arm and your triceps muscle on the back, and see how they work in tandem.

Your remaining muscles are composed of *cardiac* (myocardium) and *smooth* muscle. Cardiac, or heart, muscle is responsible for keeping your heart pumping blood throughout your body. The muscle found in your blood vessels, as well as in the walls of your stomach, intestines, uterus, and bladder, is known as smooth muscle. Among its many other functions, smooth muscle changes the diameter of blood vessels and helps substances move through the intestinal tract. Since we have no control over any of the smooth muscles, they're also known as *involuntary* muscles.

How Your Muscles Work

The skeletal muscles of your body are interesting pieces of complex, sophisticated machinery. Very efficient at turning fuel into motion, skeletal muscles grow stronger and larger through E-Centric training. Once you understand how your skeletal muscles react to the two seconds up, six seconds down way of resistance training, you will begin to get better results from your workouts.

Our muscles consist of thousands of tiny cells, each of which is connected to the brain through *motor* nerves. These nerves originate in the part of the brain called the *motor cortex,* the area that controls all of our physical movements. The motor nerve passes through the spine and branches out into a number of smaller nerves. These smaller motor nerve branches invigorate the nearby muscle cells called *fibers.*

The group of muscle cells innervated by one motor nerve is called a *motor unit.* Every time the master motor nerve sends an impulse to a muscle, the motor unit plays an important role. A motor unit in large muscles, such as the quadriceps on the front of the thigh or the hamstrings on the back of the thigh, may consist of more than a thousand individual fibers.

The first time you attempt to lift a heavy weight, the motor cortex in your brain does not know how many motor units it needs to recruit in order to lift the weight successfully. What happens then is that small sensors in the muscles let the brain know what is going on in the muscle: "Help! We're being asked to lift a heavy weight!" If the brain does not initially recruit enough muscle cells to lift the weight, these sensors instantly send a signal to recruit even more fibers. Come back another day to lift the same weight, and your central nervous system has "learned" how many fibers it needs to recruit to lift the weight smoothly.

Think of your muscle fibers as long, large cylinders, each containing *myofibrils,* which are containers of muscle proteins called *actin* and *myosin.* It's these proteins that allow the muscle cell to contract in as little as one one-thousandth of a second after the order to move is relayed from the brain.

Muscle fibers are constructed of strings of repeating units called *sarcomeres.* Think of a sarcomere as a pair of stiff hairbrushes with the bristles pushed together. The bristles are formed of two different types of filament, and each brush has only one type. One filament type has thousands of copies of myosin along its length. Myosin proteins stick out from the filament like oars from a boat. The other

The Three Types of Muscle Actions

- *Isometric.* This type of muscle action does not use weights to provide resistance, and the muscle does not change length. Instead, you oppose your muscle against an object without changing the length of the muscle. An example of an isometric exercise is pressing your two palms together in front of your chest as hard as you can. The pectoral muscles of your chest and the biceps and triceps muscles of your upper arm exert force, but their lengths do not change.
- *Concentric.* Suppose you pick up a dumbbell and perform a biceps curl by bringing it from your thigh to your chest. As you curl the weight up, your working biceps muscles contract (or shorten). This is called a *concentric* action.
- *Eccentric.* When you lower the weight, the working biceps muscles lengthen. I like to call this an E-Centric movement, and I ask that you take six seconds to lower the weight in each and every exercise that you perform. It's the E-Centric motion that stimulates the most muscle development.

filament type carries thousands of copies of actin, to which myosin sticks.

When the muscle fiber contracts, the myosin and actin act like a ratchet mechanism. The myosin changes its angle relative to the backbone of its filament, just like an oar relative to the boat it is powering. Then its bond with the actin is broken and re-formed with another actin further up the filament. The end result is a pulling together of the brushes—a muscular contraction.

How powerfully the muscle fiber can contract depends on how stretched it is, or how far apart the brushes are. As the brushes pull apart, there comes a point where the maximum force exerted during contraction begins to weaken. The number of molecules of myosin able to bond with actin becomes limited.

Researchers in Australia have discovered that this point is not reached at exactly the same time by all sarcomeres because the spacing of sarcomeres along muscle fibers is not always uniform. What happens is that the fiber begins to behave like one of those drinking straws that has a flexible section on one end to curve over the edge of a glass. If you stretch such a straw, first one bend pops, then another. Just like the straw, the muscle fiber develops areas of weakness around the sarcomeres, and where the brushes come apart, they pop: the sarcomeres have been torn, and the muscle fiber dies.

What Makes Muscles Feel Stiff?

Almost twenty-five years ago, I began investigating creatine phosphokinase (CPK), a special protein that was thought to be found only in the heart. At the time, doctors routinely used this molecule as an important cardiac marker. Whenever a person had heart disease and his or her heart tissue became damaged, cells would die and release proteins into the bloodstream. Prominent among them was CPK, and when it was abnormally elevated, that meant a heart attack had occurred.

One year, after taking muscle biopsies and other samples from a group of elite runners who had competed in the twenty-six-mile

Boston Marathon, I found that to a person their CPK levels were elevated. This was cause for concern. Was each highly trained runner unwittingly suffering from heart damage?

Upon further examination, I found that their CPK levels went up not because of any heart abnormality, but because the leg muscles of the runners had been damaged during the race. Some of the runners were actually so sore and stiff that they hobbled for many days afterward.

It has long been known that some types of exercise lead to muscle soreness, especially if you are out of shape and begin an aggressive training program. This kind of stiffness has been attributed to the buildup of lactic acid in the muscles. Some researchers had thought the soreness experienced by the marathon runners was caused by some sort of chemical problem, such as an imbalance of calcium. While lack of calcium might have contributed somewhat, it couldn't explain all of the damage that had occurred.

Reviewing the typical training of distance runners quickly led me to the source of the problem. These world-class athletes generally run anywhere from forty to sixty miles a week in their training, twice a day on nearly flat surfaces. Hills are typically avoided during workouts because they put too much stress on the body. However, a good portion of the Boston Marathon course is extremely hilly, especially "Heartbreak Hill," which runners confront between miles 20 and 21 on their way to the finish line. The racers have to work extra hard going up the steep hill, and in trying to make up for lost time they speed down the hill. This is a completely unfamiliar activity for most of them. Gravity assists them as they take extra long steps and bound down the roadway.

The runners' leg muscles are well conditioned for the normal pounding they do on level ground. But the *downhill* running in the marathon puts a tremendous stress on their quadriceps and calf muscles, which have to act as brakes to slow down each descending footfall. The end result is elevated CPK levels, plus temporary yet severe muscle damage that causes the runners to limp long after the race is over.

I suspected that the key to the elevated CPK levels and the muscle soreness had to do with the mechanics of the muscle action. Muscles are designed to contract, and most forms of muscular contraction lead to a shortening of the muscle. As I mentioned earlier, muscles that control joints are designed to work in opposing pairs. However, in running downhill, those same leg muscle fibers simultaneously stretch *and* contract. While running *up* Heartbreak Hill made the runners tired, running *down* the hill made them tired and sore because the leg muscles were being stretched *and* microscopically torn as their muscles resisted the lowering actions of the leg.

Remember the drinking straw? When sarcomeres are torn and muscle fibers die, scavenger cells in the body clean up the molecular debris. Typically you experience soreness within twenty-four to forty-eight hours.

Muscles are not regularly called upon to cope with long bouts of E-Centric exercise. When they are, the result is temporary damage, weakness, and soreness. However, to my surprise, this is actually a protective device that has several key advantages!

E-Centrics Build Better Muscle

The interesting thing I eventually found out was that just one bout of E-Centric exercise is enough to encourage the muscles to adapt and protect themselves against the next potential round of E-Centric contraction. The muscles do this not only by repairing the areas damaged by the exercise, but also by changing the entire structure of the muscle fibers and incorporating extra bits at the end. The body's response to E-Centric exercise is interesting because it seems that muscle is continually fine-tuning its own length. New muscle fiber is built to replace the old, but this new fiber packs in more sarcomeres than before. With more sarcomeres along the same length of fiber, there is less chance of stretching any one sarcomere to the point of no return. These muscles then show a greater capacity to contract when stretched. In short: they become stronger.

Studies show that rats that have been made to run *downhill* adapt to this E-Centric stress by producing up to 15 percent more sarco-

I gave up entirely on weight training in my early twenties. I didn't have any good program to follow, and I wasn't making any progress. Ten years later, AstroFit and the E-Centric way of lifting have changed all of that. I started with eight-pound dumbbells for most exercises, and at three months, I was moving twenty-pound weights with ease.

—*Laura, age 39*

meres in their thigh muscles than rats that run only *uphill*. When you lift weights, you need to "damage" the muscle to bring about growth—and E-Centric exercise causes the greatest amount of controlled damage.

Slowing Down for Rapid Gains

E-Centrics build the muscles of your upper, middle, and lower body better than anything else—and they build them fast. Unfortunately, most people don't capitalize on the all-important E-Centric half of exercises. They're into speed and trying to lift heavy weights. This is just a mind game. They're lifting weights, yes, but they're getting only half the benefit of their efforts because their muscles are not being challenged in the downward phase.

E-Centric training is slow and steady. You choose a weight you can raise and lower ten consecutive times. If you struggle to get to six or seven repetitions and can go no farther, you then use a lighter weight. Once you can do ten repetitions in perfect form, you're ready to use a heavier weight.

Performing an E-Centric exercise in the two-six cadence—two seconds up, six seconds down—prevents the "cheating" that typically comes from jerking the dumbbells up or rocking your body to raise heavy weights. Quick movements like this just exploit momentum. If you lack the strength to lower the weight slowly, you miss the all-important E-Centric phase.

Imagine you're lowering a weight in your hand. Picture the biceps

The great thing about E-Centrics is, they gave me a solid foundation for doing other things. For one, they jump-started my metabolism. I developed muscle mass while losing a great deal of body fat. My strength and energy level also went up. Now I'm into speed walking and swimming every week as well. I haven't felt this great since I was a kid.

—Maryanne, age 40

muscles of your upper arms as brakes that are slowing the weight as you bring it back to the starting position. By reducing the momentum, you make the muscle work harder against gravity. This slow, controlled descent is a challenge you will face with each and every repetition.

Try an E-Centric Exercise Right Now

To fully understand how an E-Centric works and feels, try a Level One exercise, the modified push-up. Read the directions first, then get down on an exercise mat and perform five repetitions. By starting with your arms straight, torso in the air, you will begin this exercise with the E-Centric phase.

- Get down on all fours on an exercise mat with your arms extended, palms flat on the floor, shoulder width apart, fingers pointing forward. Your feet can be straight out behind you (perpendicular to the floor) or in the air; just don't cross them, or you will put pressure on your lower back. When your arms are straight, your knees should be bent at slightly more than a ninety-degree angle.
- Slowly lower your torso to the floor, counting slowly to six. As you count, think *one–one thousand, two–one thousand, three–one thousand,* and so on. As you descend, do not hold your breath.
- Touch the mat with your chest by the sixth second.
- Pause one second.

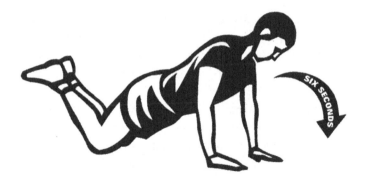

You will now begin the concentric, or upward, phase of the exercise.

- Count one-two-up. Keep your back straight, and, using your knees as the pivot point, push your torso away from the floor as you straighten your arms and rise back to the starting position.

After just five E-Centric repetitions, you undoubtedly noticed a big difference between performing an E-Centric push-up and the standard version. You probably felt tightness in the pectoral muscles of your chest and a burning sensation in your shoulder muscles as you were slowly lowering yourself. These are both signs that your muscles are being worked—perhaps for the first time.

Maximum Strength

Each muscle is a distinct, genetically determined blend of what's called *slow-twitch,* or Type I, fibers, and *fast-twitch,* or Type II, fibers. Your slow-twitch fibers are called upon during low-intensity exercise, such as bicycling and walking. When you perform E-Centrics, it's your powerful fast-twitch fibers that spring into action. The problem with fast-twitch fibers is that their numbers decline with age. If you don't use them, you lose them.

What E-Centrics do is maximally strengthen your remaining fast-twitch fibers. These fibers will be mobilized to perform the high-intensity strength-training exercises, while the slow-twitch fibers provide the endurance to perform ten repetitions of each exercise.

The progressive E-Centric program effectively maintains your fast-twitch/slow-twitch blend, beefing up the size of both types of fibers in the process. What this means is that you will be able to take on more daunting physical tasks—lifting heavier weights, pulling a heavy suitcase, pushing a lawn mower, and running up stairs—and perform them as well as or better than someone in his twenties.

An Anatomy Lesson: The Muscles of the Body

Has this recently happened to you?

- You bend over to pick up your child, and your lower back goes into a painful spasm.
- While carting in the groceries from the car to your kitchen, you don't have enough strength in your hands and a bag suddenly falls to the ground.
- Working in your garden for a few hours, turning the soil and putting in new bulbs seems easy enough, but several hours later you ache all over and have difficulty getting out of your chair.
- After sitting for hours in front of your computer monitor at work, your neck starts to ache. Walking is difficult because your legs and back are so stiff.
- Instead of walking up flights of stairs, which you know will leave you panting, you look for an elevator or escalator.

For many people, aging has to do with loss of strength and an accumulation of assorted aches and pains that result from performing the routine activities of everyday life. Although physical discomfort can come on suddenly, it may actually be the cumulative result of years of not having enough strength and flexibility in your muscles, tendons, and ligaments to perform various movements properly. This slow but steady physical debilitation and onset of pain over the years ultimately lead to accelerated aging. My message to you is that it won't be this way if you take steps right now to reverse that un-healthy trend with E-Centric training.

Let's look at the many muscles that are specifically targeted by the E-Centric exercises and their major functions. The exercises that you will be performing will train these very same muscles, leaving you strong, supple, and ready for whatever life brings your way.

Muscles of the Upper Body: Your Arms, Chest, Shoulders, and Back

When we talk about upper-body muscles, most people are quick to think that it's the biceps of the arm or the pectoral muscles of the chest that get the most exercise. But surprisingly, it's these muscles, along with the deltoids and trapezius of the shoulder and the latis-simus of the back, that are the most often ignored. The end result is an upper-body Siberia. Women are left with less-than-optimal upper body strength, while men, even those with brawny biceps developed through work or strength training, often have weak muscles in their shoulders, back, and chest. These critical upper body muscles re-spond quickly to E-Centrics.

At the back of your shoulders and neck, and descending between your shoulder blades like a large kite, are the two trapezius muscles. Their job is to draw your head back, rotate it, and help you shrug your shoulders. The deltoids, on the tops and sides of your shoulders, help lift your arms to the side, swing them back and forth, and raise them upwards. The pair of muscles called the biceps in your upper arm help lift your forearm. The three-part triceps, covering most of the back of your upper arm, oppose the biceps to help straighten the arm.

Your chest and back are supported by much larger muscles. The pectoralis major, the big muscle of your chest, moves your arms front and center and gives you the force to push. The latissimus dorsi, the largest muscles of your back, go from below each armpit all the way to the center of your back. These are the muscles that help pull your arms toward your body. The teres major and the rhomboids, which help your shoulder blades squeeze, frequently suffer from disuse and

MAJOR MUSCLES OF THE BODY

Review the major muscle groups. These are the muscles you will be working with the various E-Centric exercises. To get the most from your training, focus your attention on the muscles being exercised as you raise and lower the weights.

FRONT OF THE BODY

1. **SHOULDERS**
   Push-ups, dumbbell lateral raise, dips, lat pull-down
2. **CHEST (PECTORALS)**
   Push-ups, dumbbell chest press, dips
3. **BICEPS**
   Dumbbell curls, lat pull-down
4. **FOREARMS**
   Dumbbell curls, push-ups, dips
5. **ABDOMEN (ABS)**
   E-Centric sit-up, squat
6. **QUADRICEPS (QUADS)**
   Squat, forward lunge, leg press
7. **KNEES**
   Forward lunge, squat

BACK OF THE BODY

8. **NECK**
   Push-ups, cobra
9. **UPPER BACK**
   Lateral raise, lat pull-down
10. **TRICEPS**
    Bench dips, push-ups
11. **LOW BACK**
    Cobra, dips, squat, forward lunge
12. **BUTTOCKS (GLUTEALS)**
    Squat, forward lunge
13. **HAMSTRINGS**
    Hamstring curl, forward lunge
14. **CALVES (GASTROCNEMIUS)**
    Heel raise

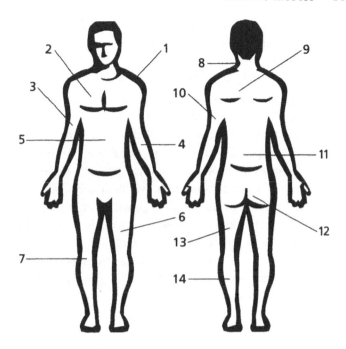

from being forced into the hunched-over position that comes from too much slouching in office chairs.

Exercising these upper-body muscles E-Centrically produces notable improvements in strength and appearance. Many of these muscles get little exercise from ordinary routines, and they respond quickly to E-Centrics. Improving the strength of your upper body muscles will also enhance your posture. Strong muscles hold your head more erect, lift your upper chest, and draw your shoulders down and back. Both men and women find that any number of daily tasks, from carrying groceries to shoveling snow to putting luggage into overhead airline bins, become much easier.

Strengthening Your Shoulders

The shoulder girdle is an intricate complex consisting of four anatomically interrelated but quite distinct joints that work together in a synchronized rhythm to permit motion. The shoulder is totally dependent for its stability, as well as its complex function, on the various muscles and ligaments that surround it.

The shoulder muscles can be divided into those that control and those that rotate the shoulder blade on the chest wall. The first group is called the parascapular muscles, and it includes the deltoid, trapezius, and pectoralis major, plus the latissimus dorsi, which comes off the back along the base of the spine. This superficial layer of muscle is responsible for big power tasks such as lifting.

The fine-tuning muscles, one layer beneath these larger power muscles, are the four rotator cuffs, which attach in a clockwise fashion around the ball of the shoulder joint. Strong, stable rotator cuff muscles allow the shoulder to remain pain-free and to function in such complex acts as serving a tennis ball.

As you get older, your risk of shoulder injuries increases. This is mainly due to uncorrected muscular imbalances, as well as to normal wear and tear, which can cause a breakdown of collagen (an important protein found in the ligaments, tendons, and cartilage). To prevent shoulder injuries, you need to maintain the strength, flexibility, and balance of all the shoulder muscles—a primary benefit of upper-body E-Centrics.

Strengthening Your Back—and Avoiding Backaches

The ability to stand and sit upright for long periods of time without discomfort depends on the spinal column. Running the length of the back from the base of the skull to the tip of the coccyx, the spinal column, or backbone, provides the body with its basic stability.

Within the spine is the spinal cord, the major nerve impulse highway that transmits messages to and from the brain. Thirty-one major nerve roots pass from the spinal cord on each side of the column—nerves that allow your muscles to contract and let you perceive various physical sensations.

Tough, fibrous ligaments, as well as muscles, extend from the skull to the sacrum. Finally, large and powerful muscles in the back contract and relax to enable you to stand and move. These are the erector spinae group, which runs along both sides of the spine from the base to the chest. This group consists of many intertwining muscles that are crucial for a strong back. The upper- and middle-body E-Centric exercises specifically target this critical area, producing the kind of posture that will make back pain a distant memory.

There's a clear reason why humans are plagued with stiff, aching backs. Sitting eight to ten hours a day—as many of us do—results in slouching and places excessive pressure on the spinal discs and soft tissues. Many backaches are due to weak muscles. It's important to note, though, that a sudden movement can trigger a backache, as can too much or too little exercise. A sedentary lifestyle exacerbates the problem, as can sleeping on a soft mattress. Pregnancy, which causes ligaments to relax, makes the joints and discs more vulnerable to damage. Poor posture and repeated bending also stress the back. A back attack can strike after as seemingly innocuous a movement as leaning over to tie your shoelace.

Eight out of ten Americans will have at least one acute episode of lower-back pain in their lives—and this statistic includes even the most fitness-conscious among us. After headaches, back discomfort is the most frequent pain complaint. It can range from seconds of annoyance to weeks of agony.

When people complain about "throwing out" their back, they usually mean their lower back. Although many back structures can cause pain, overworked or understretched muscles in the lower back are often responsible. In most cases, the muscles have weakened due to inactivity. They may have lost their elasticity because they haven't been stretched sufficiently, or they may have tightened and gone into spasm in response to stress.

Muscles of the Middle Body: Your Abdomen

A firm midsection with rippling muscles not only has aesthetic appeal but makes good physiological sense. When your abdominal muscles are strong, they work like a natural girdle that supports your internal organs and your back. Without strong abdominal muscles, you can't have a strong back or good posture.

Starting with getting out of bed in the morning, it's your abdominal muscles that play a crucial role in how you move throughout the day. Bend. Twist. Turn. Sit down. Stand up. Lift your legs. Walk. Run. With well-developed abdominals, these movements are effortless. These important muscles form what's now popularly called "the core" of the body and are at the epicenter of all movement. Many of the E-Centric exercises strengthen the abdominals, both directly and indirectly.

The abdominal muscles begin just below the ribs and extend down to slightly below the navel. They consist of four layers of overlapping fibers that crisscross the lower ribs, pelvis, and abdominal cavity diagonally, horizontally, and vertically. Their primary functions are to support the lower back, provide movement to the trunk, and keep the internal organs in place.

The rectus abdominis is the long, flat muscle on the front of the torso that makes it appear as if your muscles were rippled. The external and internal obliques are the large muscles running along the front and sides of the abdomen that give definition to the waistline. And the transversus abdominis helps with breathing.

Avoiding Belly Bulge

Even the strongest abdominal muscles can't hold in a potbelly, no matter how hard you work them. The abdominal area is a major site for storing excess body fat in both men and women. No matter how many E-Centric sit-ups or squats you do, when you're overweight, the fat covers the abdominal muscles. There is no such thing as "spot

---

The body fat had begun to accumulate around my waist by the time I was twenty-five. I used to run a few times a week, but all those miles did nothing for my potbelly. With the E-Centrics, I started to notice a difference by my twelfth workout. By three months I was in my old jeans and running faster, too.

—Richard, age 32

reducing" and losing your potbelly by performing only abdominal exercises. The appearance of any area of the body depends on a combination of factors, including diet, exercise, and heredity. When you perform E-Centrics for the full twelve weeks, you will build calorie-hungry tissue that will help reduce your overall body fat percentage. As the fat is pared off from your entire body over time, you will eventually lose the fat from your midsection.

Muscles of the Lower Body: Your Legs and Hips

The largest muscles, and most likely the ones in your body that are the best developed right now, are found in your lower body. Your legs and hips support and move your body, which, in the case of most adults, means moving more than 100 pounds regularly during the course of a day.

Your largest lower-body muscle is your gluteus maximus, which covers both buttocks. Its main job is to help straighten the legs from your hips, such as when you stand up from a chair. The quadriceps, four-part muscles, are the principal shapers of your thighs and supply much of the power in forward movement by straightening your legs from your knees. These muscles are used whenever you jump, run, kick, lift, or push. Strengthening your "quads" also makes it easier to lift objects the safe way—with your legs, rather than your back, providing most of the strength.

On the backs of your thighs, the hamstrings, three-part muscles, oppose the quadriceps and help bend the knees. Many people ignore their hamstrings when strength training, overdeveloping their quadriceps to such an extent that they can easily tear their hamstring muscle when the quadriceps contract to help them run or jump.

The big muscles in your calf, the gastrocnemius and the soleus, join at the Achilles tendon fixed to your heel. These muscles pull on your heel, allowing you to rise on your toes as you walk or run.

Protecting Your Knees

The knees are subjected to many stresses. When you walk, the knees cushion the equivalent of up to 1.5 times your body weight. Landing from a jump causes knee stress to skyrocket. To hurt your knee, all you have to do is slip on a stair, take a tumble on icy pavement, or walk for extended periods in high-heeled shoes. Being overweight strains the knee joints, too.

The quadriceps are vitally important to the knees, which are vulnerable to injury. Knees are not built to rotate. Although this provides great stability to the lower body, it exposes the knee to danger whenever forces come from the wrong direction. By strengthening your quadriceps, you reinforce and protect your knees from injury. However, don't let the outer quadriceps muscles become stronger than the muscles in your inner thighs. When this happens, the kneecap no longer tracks normally and walking down stairs produces pain.

People who don't exercise much suffer many knee injuries. Years of sitting with knees flexed at a ninety-degree angle, without much movement, wear down the cartilage under the kneecap, producing pain and inflammation. Inactivity and advancing age can also lead to loss of important leg muscles and subsequent misalignment of the knees.

Strengthening your leg muscles with E-Centrics will greatly benefit your knees. Exercising the quadriceps and hamstrings, as well as reinforcing the muscles of the inner thighs, is crucial. Maintaining strength and flexibility allows you to maintain a maximum range of

---

My knees were hurting for the past four years, so much so that I started to limp. My wife said that I was acting like I was eighty. With the increase in strength after the first week of E-Centrics, I found that I wasn't limping any more. And my wife has even said that I'm starting to move around like I used to.

—*John, age 54*

---

knee motion and fully lubricates the knee joint. Stronger, more flexible muscles can also provide protection to the knee cartilage that supports the integrity of the ligaments. The more powerful and more supple your leg muscles are, the more stable your knees will be.

Are You Ready?

Now that you know something about your body and how weak muscles can lead to discomfort and disability, making you feel old long before your time, it's time to make the decision to do something about it. Even if you've avoided exercise or have never lifted weights, think of all the benefits you'll get once you begin. Not only will you look and feel better, but your muscles will finally work together to effortlessly support you in everything that you do throughout the day.

4

The Keys to Training Success

The world belongs to the energetic.
—RALPH WALDO EMERSON

I was settled into my aisle seat and looking over some study results on my laptop while waiting for the other Little Rock–bound passengers to board. Returning from a two-day meeting with NASA officials in Washington, D.C., I was fatigued and was looking forward to being able to stretch out a bit on the flight once we were airborne.

I was lucky. The two seats next to me were vacant, and people kept moving past to other seats in the back of the plane. But then a harried-looking road warrior with an overstuffed carry-on bag came down the aisle. His eyes were focused on one of the empty spots in my row. Silver-haired and breathing heavily, he looked as if he'd had a very long day.

"Excuse me, but I have the window seat in there," he said. I stood up and let him squeeze past. As he eased into his seat, he let out a weary "Oomph!"

"The body just doesn't work like it did when you were twenty-five, that's for sure," he announced to me as he was forcing his carry-on under the seat in front of him. He finally gave the bag a strong kick with his foot to wedge it out of sight.

My new traveling companion squirmed as he tried to adjust his bulk comfortably into the small coach seat. He wiped the droplets of perspiration off his brow with a cocktail napkin that I handed to him. "The escalator was out, and I had to race up the stairs," he explained. It was clear that this man was in the throes of a personal physical fitness battle that had gotten out of hand. His cheeks were flushed, and his chest was still rising and falling rapidly. "When you get to be my age, the body just isn't the same. I used to be in great shape," he said. "But once you reach forty-five, you put on the weight, and it's downhill from there!"

The Mind/Body Connection

Once we were aloft and my traveling companion was dozing, I thought about the various factors that have an impact on aging. What makes us "old"? Chronological age has nothing to do with it. I've seen spry eighty-year-olds bouncing on trampolines with their grandchildren, seventy-year-olds finishing the Boston Marathon way ahead of thirty-year-olds, and sixty-five-year-olds flashing across the finish line of the Ironman Triathlon in Hawaii. Our age in years has nothing to do with how old we are, how we feel, and what we can accomplish. However, not being in optimal physical condition is certainly a major determinant, which was quite obvious in my seatmate. Not maintaining fitness and health for the longest possible time increases the odds of dying earlier.

Aging well is all about attitude, regular exercise, and a dogged persistence to keep at it every day of the week. Mind and body are inseparable, and being in good physical shape can certainly enhance your feelings of optimism and overall vitality.

I recalled a recent study that was presented at the annual meeting of the American College of Sports Medicine that touched on that very important issue. Researchers from Johns Hopkins University found that older folks who were in good shape and have a relatively low body fat percentage also seemed to have a better outlook on life than those who were less active and less lean.

The study looked at thirty-six people in their fifties, sixties, and seventies who signed up for an exercise program. Other than having mild hypertension, the volunteers were extremely healthy. The researchers then calculated the participants' fitness levels from a treadmill test, recorded their muscle strength during weight-lifting exercises, and measured their percentages of body fat. The volunteers then completed two questionnaires regarding their mental health and mood. The researchers found that the volunteers who were more fit were less tired, less depressed, less angry, less tense, and in an overall better mood.

Contrary to anything else you may have heard, you're never too old to exercise, improve yourself, and make physical gains. Remember my eighty- and ninety-year-old friends who took part in my strength-training research? They made gains in muscle strength and endurance that I would have expected from people thirty or forty years younger.

Commit yourself to improvement by starting your fitness program today. Stick with it, and on your next birthday I guarantee that instead of feeling a year older, you'll feel several years younger.

Make Time for Exercise

How can you fit exercise into your busy schedule? According to the latest national figures, only one in four adults follows through with the recommended thirty minutes of exercise most days of the week. Although most say that they understand the value of exercise and how it can help relieve stress and prolong life, many nonexercisers say they are simply too busy and don't have enough time. With Americans watching an average of four hours of TV daily, having no time for exercise is not a good enough excuse.

Let's take a closer look at the time element and see how it actually breaks down for most people. Out of the 168 hours in a week, you spend on average forty to fifty hours working and fifty or so sleeping. Simple math leaves you with sixty-eight "free" hours. I ask that you make a commitment to set aside at least three of them for physical activity. Make getting in shape your number one priority for the next three months, and let those three hours be a gift to yourself each and every week.

I know personal workouts can be difficult to schedule, but they're imperative. Like you, I have similar obligations and not a lot of free time. But I know the power of exercise, and I appreciate all the great feelings I get from a mere thirty minutes of physical activity. It's not that I have more willpower than you. I really don't think I do. What I do have is an exercise habit. I've established a routine of daily exercise, just like making my bed, brushing my teeth, and combing my hair in the morning. And regular exercise is a habit I happen to enjoy.

It's amazing how people can transform themselves with a simple exercise program. I'm constantly impressed when I go to the gym in my research lab and see people who didn't look like much twelve months before—a little too heavy in most cases, with sloppy posture and poorly defined musculature—looking revitalized. Many had complained of back problems or assorted aches and pains, and of not being able to sleep well. But over the course of the year, without fail, something wonderful happened to each one. They've been able to gradually transform themselves into the picture of health and vitality by hoisting dumbbells and using the various pieces of exercise equipment in the lab. It takes commitment to bring about this kind of transformation, but through persistence that's exactly what these people have done.

The surprising thing you will discover about exercise is that it actually creates *more* time in your day. You'll feel better and have more energy, so you'll become more effective in your work and get more things done. Once you begin exercising, you may find that you get up earlier, stay up later, and feel more energetic throughout the day.

When Is the Best Time to Exercise?

Is it the first thing in the morning, before you sip that first steaming cup of coffee? Or is the best time right after dinner, so you can work off that extra helping of roast beef? When the best time is really comes down to a question of consistency. At what time of day are the odds consistently stacked in your favor that you will exercise? Find that time, and most of the battle is won.

Make exercise a priority. You *can* find the time to exercise. Try to find the optimum time available to you each day, with the least chance for interruption or schedule changes. Only when you exercise consistently will you have something that's truly beneficial for your heart and your soul. Only then will exercise become a habit.

Morning

If you happen to be a morning person, you have a big advantage over late-day exercisers, as there's a better chance you'll make exercise a daily habit by doing it early in the day. Studies have shown that people who exercise in the morning are more likely to stick with their exercise programs.

- *Advantages:* Your phone won't be chirping, and there aren't too many meetings you will need to attend or any other kinds of distraction shortly after dawn. In addition, after a night's sleep, you've used up your carbohydrate stores and your body has switched to burning body fat as a fuel as you exercise. Get the workout out of the way, and you'll be energized right through to bedtime. When you're finished, you don't have to think about your workout again all day.
- *Disadvantages:* After hitting the snooze alarm twice, it's too easy to take an exercise pass for the entire day.

The Middle of the Day

Exercising in the middle of the day can be difficult logistically, but your body will love it. You can perform the E-Centric exercises that don't require weights right in your office.

- *Advantages:* A great work break. At midday, muscle strength is greatest and energy is peaking. The "exercise high" you get will carry over through the afternoon.
- *Disadvantages:* Meetings. Lunch. Fatigue. Crowded gym facilities. Plus you need to shower and then put your work clothes back on.

I tried various exercise programs over the past ten years. I felt good after my workouts, but nothing compares to how I feel after the E-Centric dumbbell program. I sleep better than ever, and I'm usually up before my alarm goes off, wide awake and ready for a new day.

—Liz, age 33

After Work

Exercising after work allows you to take care of all your work obligations first. The problem is that your "to do" list may not have any perceptible end.

- *Advantages:* Exercising later shakes off the lethargy and the pent-up stresses of the day and gives you a good chance to get pumped up. The workout also prepares you for a nice night's sleep.
- *Disadvantages:* Fatigue. Family obligations. Crowded gym facilities. When you've already had a long day, it's more tempting to skip your workout.

Late Evening

Exercising in the late evening is another option. Whether this works for you or not is very individual. After exercising, some people fall asleep in minutes after their head hits the pillow, while others find it difficult to get to sleep right away.

- *Advantages:* You clear your mind and work the stress of the day out of your body before bed.
- *Disadvantages:* If you have a family, they want to be with you. If you're really tired, you may decide that working out is too much effort.

Keep Your Eyes on the Prize

Often exercise isn't easy, even for regular exercisers like myself. There are days when I'm tired and I'd like to be doing anything other than lifting weights or riding my bike. And so I push myself. Five to ten minutes into the workout, I'm usually feeling better, more inspired, and ready to take on the world. When you're committed to your exercise program, no matter what difficulty is presented, no matter how tired you feel, deep inside you know that what you'll get from your exercise far exceeds the rewards from anything else you could be doing.

I've always believed that exercise is a celebration of life and an endorsement of good health. Whenever you make the time to exercise, you are celebrating life at its best. Therefore, my question to you is straightforward: Are you ready to make the commitment to becoming physically active on a daily basis? By this I mean, are you ready to take up the thirty- to forty-five-minute daily exercise program I've devised for you? Not only will it make you sweat, shape your body, and pare off fat, but it will also help reduce your stress levels and make you feel great all over.

Many people read about exercise and scientific breakthroughs, yet they do nothing with that important information. This reminds me of the riddle of the two frogs. One day, two frogs were sitting on a lily pad and one of them decided to jump into the water. How many were left sitting on the lily pad?

The correct answer is two. That's because deciding to jump and actually jumping are two different things.

The moral here is that you will improve yourself only when you act upon what you've learned. You must be willing to take that step forward and put all that accumulated knowledge into action. Start today.

Over the past two decades, I've worked with thousands of people who have succeeded in becoming strong and fit. Along the way, I've identified six important steps that have helped them achieve their personal best. I ask that you learn from those who've already succeeded. Do what they've done, and I guarantee that you'll accomplish similar results. Don't *decide* to do it—*do it.*

Making exercise a permanent part of your life has to do with setting goals and then maintaining your motivation over months. Here's the six-step program I want you to follow on your way to becoming a new, fit, healthier you.

AstroFit Step 1: Set Your Personal Goals

Understand that one of the most difficult aspects of working out is that you often have to be your own coach, inspiration, and motivating force. That being the case, take the time to *write down* both the short-term and long-term goals that you want to achieve from the exercise program.

You may be thinking, why should I do this? Simply because it helps provide direction and makes it real. Would you think of getting into your car without a planned destination and then drive aimlessly until you ran out of gas? Unfortunately, that's just what too many people do when they begin an exercise program. They have no compass or map—which is what written goals provide—and eventually they give up.

Here's the best way to keep you interested and focused in your exercise. List on a sheet of paper all of your short-term aspirations. Make them exciting and challenging but attainable. Short-term goals are important because they serve to bolster your spirits, motivate you, and encourage you to continue with your program. These goals should be attainable in one to twelve months. Some of these short-term goals can include:

- Exercising two or three times a week
- Losing ten pounds of body weight in eight weeks
- Losing two inches from your waistline or hips
- Being able to walk/jog two miles without stopping
- Going from one to two sets of repetitions per exercise
- Lowering your resting pulse five beats
- Walking up two flights of stairs without getting winded
- Adding two inches of muscle to your chest, arms, or legs
- Cutting back or eliminating smoking and drinking

Long-term goals are also important and should be attainable in at least one year to eighteen months. Write down your long-term goals, too. Some examples are:

- Exercising daily
- Losing thirty pounds
- Paring off 10 percent of your body fat
- Gaining ten pounds of muscle
- Decreasing your clothing size
- Making the "spare tire" around your waistline disappear
- Dropping a minute off your mile jogging time
- Increasing your bench press by fifty pounds
- Competing in a 5K fun run
- Completing a century (100-mile) bike ride

Goal setting is important if you are serious about continuing your exercise program. The sooner you define, write down, and verbalize what you really want from your AstroFit program, the sooner you'll be on your way to achieving your aims.

Lasting fitness won't be achieved overnight, but it will come through regular weekly workouts of at least thirty minutes per session. Be patient with the AstroFit program. When you're consistent in your approach to exercise, you will soon start to see some significant changes in both how you feel and how you look.

AstroFit Step 2: Engage in Positive Self-Talk

Exercise professionals agree with me when I say that it takes at least two months for exercise to become a regular health habit. And it all begins with "training" the mind. In the first few weeks of the AstroFit program, whenever you find that you're losing the urge to work out, try to use positive affirmations such as "I feel great when I'm exercising!" "I enjoy moving!" "When it's over I feel so relaxed!" or "I'm so much closer to getting two months under my belt" or "I'm going to achieve my goals!"

Here's my bottom line when it comes to exercise: *Other than illness and injury, there are very few valid reasons not to stick to your workout routine.* Have zero tolerance for the self-defeating thoughts that can keep you from exercising.

I've compiled a shortlist of some of the most common excuses for not exercising, along with some ways you can easily overcome them:

- *I'm too tired.* If you're really fatigued, begin your workout with the intent of completing only half of it. Once you get going, your energy level may spike and you'll find you can ease through to the end.
- *My back hurts.* If your back is sore (and your doctor has cleared you for activity), head for the swimming pool and do some gentle water aerobics. The buoyancy of the water will gently massage your back as you go through range-of-motion movements.
- *I'm expecting a phone call.* If you must receive a call, schedule it before or after your workout. And make appointments for home repairs at times that won't interfere with your exercise plans. If you're expecting a package, leave a note authorizing the delivery person to leave the parcel at the door.
- *It upsets my stomach to exercise after I eat.* Consider making exercise the very first thing you do after you wake up. If you're hungry when it's time to exercise, try a light snack such as half an apple or a piece of toast to tide you over.
- *I have to travel to another city.* Going on the road for an extended business trip should by no means spell an end to your exercise program. Most large hotels now have fitness facilities on-site; others have agreements with nearby gyms. Rubber stretch cords sold in most fitness shops fit easily into your travel kit and are an excellent "filler" for when you can't pump iron, allowing you to work out in your hotel room whenever you like.
- *I'm caught in a time squeeze.* Break up your workout day. Go for a walk or run in the morning and hit the weights in the afternoon or evening. If you're cooped up in the office all day, close your door and do some of the weightless E-Centrics.
- *Why bother? I'm not getting results.* Be patient. You are guaranteed to see and feel results if you work out consistently and follow the AstroFit diet suggestions later in this book.

- *I'm too old.* Your body is meant to move, and it's never too late to exercise. After a few weeks, with your increased endurance, strength, and flexibility, you'll feel years younger.

AstroFit Step 3: Draw Up a Contract with Someone Else

Write down the specifics of your exercise goals—for example, working out three to five days a week for thirty minutes at a time. Make the contract binding. Sign it with family or friends as witnesses. Your contract will help reinforce your resolve to follow through with your commitment to the "good" life. You can even include weekly "penalties" for missing days, such as making a contribution to your favorite charity or performing a household chore. Check in weekly with your witnesses to report on how you did.

Don't become a weekend warrior. Marathon weekend training sessions can easily lead to extreme fatigue, muscle soreness, or, worse, an injury of some sort. However, if you know beforehand that your workweek will be busier than usual, use Saturday and Sunday as two of your regular exercise days, leaving you with one weekday slot to fill.

There is a delicate balance between a firm commitment to exercise and a rigid compulsion about keeping to a predetermined workout schedule. By developing a flexible, healthy attitude about your exercise program—making it *part* of your life, not your *entire* life—your enthusiasm for exercising will always remain high.

AstroFit Step 4: Find a Workout Partner

Finding a workout partner is a way to make sure that you exercise regularly—and that you have fun doing it. Just be sure to choose wisely, so that both you and your partner will benefit. Your spouse or significant other could be your partner, but don't choose this option if you will be inclined to see his or her encouragement as nagging.

It's all a mind game if you happen to miss a workout. You have to get the idea out of your head that if you don't exercise, you're a slob or a "bad" person. You should never feel guilty about missing any workout. I'm not the disciplined exerciser that I once was, and occasionally I'll miss a day. However, whenever I do, I get fired up to work out the next day because I know how much pleasure it will bring me.

—*John Howard, three-time U.S. Olympic cyclist*

A workout partner can help you overcome embarrassment. Often, when you're just beginning to work out, especially at a fitness center or health club, it's easy to feel intimidated, either by other people who seem to be in better shape than you or by the facility itself, which might seem as though it's filled with serious "hardbodies." You and your partner can help each other get through this brief period of feeling awkward or out of place. Working together, the two of you can also keep each other motivated by challenging and encouraging each other to pursue your respective exercise goals.

It's important to be somewhat selective in choosing your partner. Find someone close to your fitness level. That way it will be easier for both of you to stay motivated and feel as though you're both making progress. Also, look for someone who shares some of your interests and values. Having some common bonds with your partner will give you lots of things to talk about while you're working out. And, if you have a particularly busy schedule and can't always find one-on-one time with a close friend, choosing to exercise together does double duty, letting you socialize and exercise at the same time.

AstroFit Step 5: Reward Yourself Frequently

Your persistence will yield results, and one of the ways of acknowledging this is by treating yourself whenever you reach one of your exercise goals. A month of workouts, for example, can equal new clothes, an upgrade in equipment, a massage, a half hour with that "hot" trainer, a yoga or Pilates class, a fancy pair of cross-trainers, a first-run movie, a night on the town, or a weekend spa getaway. You get the idea. Splurge. You've earned it.

AstroFit Step 6: Refuel with Whey and Soy

Exercise depends on proper nutrition, which gives you the energy to perform your workouts. Drinking whey or soy protein shakes before or after you exercise will provide you with everything your muscles need to repair themselves and grow.

Whey, a by-product of cheese production, contains a variety of proteins and large amounts of milk sugar, called lactose. It also has an even better amino acid profile than the highly regarded egg white. In addition, whey protein contains the highest concentration (23 to 25 percent) of branched-chain amino acids of any single protein source. This is important to exercisers because branched-chain amino acids are an integral part of muscle metabolism and are the first amino acids sacrificed during intense exercise and muscle breakdown.

Consuming soy protein (soy milk, tofu, isolated soy protein)— which is high in phytoestrogens, low in saturated fat, and a source of omega-3 fatty acids—is another easy way to meet your daily protein requirements, as well as help reduce your cholesterol levels. (*Note:* Chapters 13 and 14 discuss AstroFit nutrition in depth.)

A Checklist That Could Save Your Life

Before you embark on the AstroFit exercise program, I want you to make sure it's safe for you to exercise. If you haven't had a physical exam in the last two years, schedule a checkup. Ask yourself the following ten questions. If you answer "yes" to any of them, consult your physician, even if you're young and healthy.

* Have you experienced any pain or discomfort in the chest or surrounding area, particularly during exercise?
* Do you develop any chest pain or discomfort radiating down your arm during exercise that goes away after your workout?
* Do you ever become dizzy or faint, particularly during exercise?
* Do you have unaccustomed shortness of breath during a workout?
* Do you become nauseated during exercise?
* Have you been told by your physician that you have a heart murmur?
* Has any family member died suddenly before the age of thirty-five?
* Has a physician ever recommended that you not participate in vigorous activity or sports?
* Is there a history of coronary artery disease (heart attack, bypass surgery, angina) in your immediate family?
* Do you smoke or have high blood pressure, high cholesterol, or diabetes?

If you have any warning signs, your doctor can perform an exhaustive battery of tests to detect the presence of any cardiac abnormality.

5

Fitness by the Numbers

A goal is a dream that has an ending.
—DUKE ELLINGTON

Numbers don't lie—or do they? It would be impossible to track your progress, determine your body fat percentage, or understand your metabolism without first crunching some numbers. Because some test results are more accurate or more significant than others, this chapter will help you recognize and interpret the most important numbers you need to follow.

Understanding Metabolism

"At one time it seemed as if I could eat anything I wanted and never gain a pound," said Julie, one of my test subjects, remembering her days back in high school as an All-Sectional softball player and a world-class calorie furnace. Now age thirty-four, Julie no longer works out as she used to, and she's carrying twenty pounds more than she did during her high school glory days. Reducing her exercise regularity over the years from daily to infrequent had caused a drop-off in Julie's overall muscle mass. In the sixteen years since she had graduated from high school, Julie's loss of calorie-burning muscle, coupled with the same level of eating, had been responsible for her subsequent gain in girth.

The culprit—as I pointed out to Julie—is called *basal metabolism.* It's also called *resting metabolic rate,* or RMR. Some researchers refer to it as BMR, which is short for *basal metabolic rate.* What you need to know is that "basal" means at baseline, relaxed or resting; "metabolism" refers to the chemical processes in your body that provide energy for the maintenance of life; and "basal metabolism" basically means how fast your body uses calories to maintain the function of vital organs such as your brain, heart, liver, lungs, and kidneys. Your metabolism, which is measured in the lab as the number of calories per minute per kilogram of body weight you use, is lowest upon awakening and highest during vigorous activities.

Your basal metabolic rate accounts for 70 percent of your daily calories, which proves that almost everyone uses more energy just living than they ever do while exercising. (The exception is Tour de France bike racers, who ride anywhere from 50 to 150 miles a day for twenty-three days and consume 8,000 calories per day to keep up the pace.) But here is an interesting point: *One pound of fat burns about 2 calories per day. One pound of muscle burns as many as 50 calories per day.* You readily boost your BMR when you pack on muscle and lose fat, keeping your metabolic fires stoked to the maximum.

Between the ages of twenty and forty, an inactive person can easily gain seven or more pounds of fat, lose seven pounds of muscle, and develop a 7 percent slower metabolic rate, even though his or her weight stays exactly the same! Does the bathroom scale lie? Not exactly. But it certainly does not tell the whole story.

Basal metabolism can vary considerably from one person to another. In general, large people tend to burn more calories than smaller people do, and people with large muscles burn calories faster than people of equal weight but with a larger proportion of body fat. For example, Jenny, a five-foot-eleven, 165-pound woman with a lean and muscular build, uses more calories just by sitting in her easy chair reading the newspaper than Susan, who is five feet tall and weighs 190 pounds. Jenny's muscles require more calories, while Susan's higher percentage of body fat needs very few calories.

Many people believe that your metabolism drops as you age, making you more susceptible to weight gain. It's true that the basal metabolic rate tends to decrease starting at about age thirty, but this decline stems from a loss of muscle rather than from the aging process itself. Generally, people lose about 2 percent of their lean body mass per decade after age thirty. *The drop in basal metabolic rate is almost entirely due to a drop in muscle mass directly attributable to physical inactivity.*

Your metabolism doesn't have to drop, and you don't need to gain body fat. Follow my program and maintain lean body mass and you should have very few changes in your metabolism—at least until you reach your seventies, eighties, or beyond.

The Great Diet Paradox

At first glance, it would seem plausible that sticking to a calorie-reduced diet would help pare unwanted fat and padding from your midsection and other parts of your body. Unfortunately, dieting alone isn't enough. That's because restricted eating causes an accompanying breakdown of muscle, which is what is needed to burn fat in the first place. Also, when you reduce your caloric intake, less food is available as fuel for your daily energy needs, so you feel fatigued, with little energy to spare. In addition, your body compensates by becoming more efficient, *lowering* your metabolic rate.

Why 30 Calories Can Make a Difference

Let's say you follow the AstroFit program, laying on the muscle and burning calories. Great! Each pound of muscle burns about 15 calories a day, so if you add two pounds of muscle, you'll burn off an additional 30 calories a day. This may not seem like a lot, but over the course of a year, if you burn just an extra 30 calories a day, you'll pare three pounds from your frame. Stay inactive, however, and you will add three pounds of fat in the same time period. Over the span of a decade, that's an additional 30 pounds!

Between the ages of thirty and seventy, most people experience a loss of 20 to 30 percent of their total number of muscle cells. Two things trigger this. First, the nerves connecting the spinal cord to the muscles begin to deteriorate with age. Second, as people use their muscles less, they simply begin to atrophy from disuse.

The secret to transforming your aging body into a fat-burning machine is E-Centrics. As Julie and countless others who have followed the AstroFit prescription have found for themselves, E-Centrics will build enough muscle mass to stoke your metabolic fires so that age-related weight gain will be stopped and even reversed—without the need ever to go on a diet again.

How to Raise Your Metabolic Rate

The best way to increase your metabolic rate is to decrease the amount of fat you're carrying and replace it with muscle. This calls for a combination of muscle-building E-Centric weight workouts, some heart-pumping aerobic activity, and sensible eating. In one study I conducted, volunteers who performed strength-training exercises three times a week for three months added three pounds of metabolically active muscle. To their delight, they had to consume 15 percent more calories just to maintain their body weight! Such dramatic results occur because muscles continue to burn calories, even when you're sleeping. *Muscle is your body's engine. The bigger the engine, the more fuel you need to keep it going.*

In the AstroFit program, the aim is not to lose weight but to lose fat and gain muscle. If you're able to accomplish this, you're well on your way to achieving your antiaging goals.

Facts About Fat

Everyone needs body fat, but too much can lead to medical problems and have a negative impact on longevity. Most of us have too much body fat. It makes our clothing tight, restricts our mobility, and makes us feel uncomfortable. Being obese can trigger myriad health problems, ranging from high blood pressure and arthritis to diabetes and even cancer.

Fat, the yellowish globules layered under the skin and packed around your organs, is energy in reserve that's stored within your body for times of trauma, extremes of physical activity, reproduction, and famine. Having the proper amount of body fat contributes to your attractiveness. It provides your body with unique contours and keeps your hair glossy and your skin smooth.

When you begin to regularly consume more calories than your body burns up through activity, you slowly add to your body fat stores. To put it simply, you become fat. It doesn't happen overnight, but the longer you remain inactive, the fatter you become.

Why Fat Is So Hard to Lose

What happens when you panic at your scale weight, go on a crash diet, and begin to deprive yourself of calories in order to cut back on your body fat? Fat cells immediately mobilize to protect your body, a survival mechanism left over from more primitive times that was designed to help our prehistoric ancestors conserve fat stores when food was scarce—which was a good deal of the time. Once the fat cells detect that your caloric intake has been restricted, the production of lipogenic enzymes, used to store fat, is increased, while the production of lipolytic enzymes, used to release fat as fuel, is dramatically slowed. Your body is protecting the fat stores and letting go of even less fat to be used as body fuel. At the same time, your muscle cells begin to starve and wither, which accounts for some of the weakness and fatigue people typically experience on crash diets—and also explains why these people are just too tired to exercise.

Since fat weighs less than lean muscle tissue—muscle, bone, and your vital organs—you'd think it would be easier to lose. Not so, as too many of us already know from bitter experience. The reason for this is that body fat is the richest energy source in the body, packing a whopping 9 calories into every gram. On the other hand, carbohydrates and proteins have only 4 calories per gram. Therefore, to lose body fat, you need to burn it off. The best way to achieve this goal is to follow the AstroFit strength-training program and eating plan.

Muscle Matters Most

One of the hallmarks of extended NASA space missions has been the changing body composition of the astronauts. For reasons that are not yet entirely understood, most astronauts *lose* weight during their period in microgravity. This is likely linked to a combination of motion sickness, monotonous food choices, and a very busy work schedule. Researchers are currently working at trying to stop this weight loss because as weight plummets, so does muscle power.

Decreased food intake *accelerates* the loss of muscle tissue. On Earth, weight loss programs that include no strategies for conserving muscle cause a substantial loss of lean muscle tissue. For example, for every three pounds of fat that you lose during a *diet-alone* weight loss program, you lose one pound of muscle. Not only is this unhealthy and unwelcome, but the loss of muscle depresses your basal metabolic rate, making it even more difficult to lose weight.

Performing E-Centrics increases your lean body mass. This is important because your basal metabolic rate goes up in direct proportion to your lean body mass. Muscles burn about 25 percent of total calories, so the more lean muscle mass you have, the higher your metabolic rate—and the easier it is for you to maintain a desirable body fat level.

How Fat Are You?

Your overall body composition—where the fat is located, how much there is, and how much of your body is hard muscle—is a better measure of health and fitness than body weight alone. It used to be that the bathroom scale was all we had to let us know if we were too fat. Bathroom scales don't lie, but they provide us with only a very small part of our overall health picture. The major drawback of the scale is

Quick Fat Check

In the privacy of your room, stand naked in front of a full-length mirror and give your body a close look from head to toes. Do you look fat? Does your belly protrude? Do your buttocks droop or appear to be large? Is your chest flabby? Do the backs of your arms jiggle? Do you have "love handles"? A positive response to any of these questions means you have some work to do.

Before you put your clothes back on, I want you to jog slowly in place for fifteen seconds, lifting your feet just two to three inches off the ground as you swing your arms back and forth. What's bouncing up and down as you jog? If there's a lot of movement, it's fat.

If you don't like what you see, think of it this way: the worse you look now, the happier you'll be with your AstroFit results in just a short time!

that while it tells you how much you weigh, it's unable to tell you how *fat* you are.

Since overall body weight is all you get from your scale, you would do better to set your scale aside for the next three months. In its place, consider the following four specific steps that will help you to document your progress in the AstroFit program accurately:

1. Determine your body fat percentage.
2. Determine your body mass index (BMI).
3. Take nine circumference measurements.
4. Have someone take full-body photographs of you in a bathing suit.

1. Determine Your Body Fat Percentage

When you lower your body fat to safe levels through resistance training, you can help prevent or control the development of many life-threatening diseases. You can also help reverse the effects of aging. To calculate your percentage of body fat, you need to measure the proportion of fat and lean tissue in your body. This will give you a much better assessment of your fitness than the weight registered on your scale. A low body fat percentage also directly reflects the intensity of your training.

Generally, body fat percentages fall between 9 and 19 percent for an active man and between 14 and 25 percent for an active woman. For those of you who want to chart your body fat regularly and get very accurate measurements, Appendix A lists six popular methods based on their precision, listing them in order from the most to the least desirable.

Once you determine your body fat percentage, write this figure on the AstroFit Chart on page 84. Measure and record your body fat again at Week 4, Week 8, and Week 12.

In lieu of spending any money for special equipment for measuring body fat loss, you can easily make a fairly accurate assessment using a cloth measuring tape.

By taking various measurements on Day 1 and then comparing them at Week 4, Week 8, and Week 12 you will have a very clear idea that your body fat percentage is dropping as your muscle mass increases. See "Take Nine Circumference Measurements" on page 86 for the body parts to measure.

2. Determine Your Body Mass Index (BMI)

Your body mass index measures the relationship of your weight to your height. Determining your BMI is easy. You can let your computer do the math for you by entering your vital statistics into BMI charts on Internet health sites, such as www.consumer.gov/weightloss/bmi.htm. You also can use a calculator for the math and follow these steps:

Step 1: Weigh yourself without clothing and divide the number of pounds by 2.2. This will give you your weight in kilograms.

Step 2: Measure your height in stocking feet and divide the number of inches by 39.4. This will give you your height in meters. Multiply the number you get by itself.

AstroFit Chart

	DAY 1	WEEK 4	WEEK 8	WEEK 12

YOUR BODY
FAT PERCENTAGE

YOUR BODY
MASS INDEX

YOUR BODY
MEASUREMENTS:
   NECK
   SHOULDERS
   CHEST
   WAIST
   HIPS
   THIGH
   CALF
   UPPER ARM
   FOREARM

MUSCULAR
ENDURANCE TESTS:
   THE WALL SIT
   THE ABDOMINAL HOLD
   THE PUSH-UP

AEROBIC
ENDURANCE TEST:
   THE STEP-UP

FLEXIBILITY TEST:
   THE SIT-REACH

How Do You Measure Up?

The desirable BMI range for men is 21.9 to 22.4, and for women, 21.3 to 22.1. Between 25.1 and 30 is considered overweight. The risk of diabetes, hypertension, heart disease, and death goes up as your body mass index increases above 25. A reading over 30 is considered obese.

Height	Women Body Weight (lbs.)	Men Body Weight (lbs.)
4'10"	119	143
4'11"	124	148
5'0"	128	153
5'1"	132	158
5'2"	136	164
5'3"	141	169
5'4"	145	174
5'5"	150	180
5'6"	155	186
5'7"	159	191
5'8"	164	197
5'9"	169	203
5'10"	174	207
5'11"	179	215
6'0"	184	221
6'1"	189	227
6'2"	194	233
6'3"	200	240
6'4"	205	246
	BMI = 25	BMI = 30

Note: Men who are very muscular may have a high BMI. If you're a muscular athlete and suspect that your greater-than-ideal weight is not a problem, record only body fat percentage on your AstroFit Chart.

Step 3: Divide the result of step 1 by the result of step 2. The result. you get is your BMI.

3. Take Nine Circumference Measurements

There is nothing like before-and-after circumference measurements to let you know how well your training is going—and how much body fat is being replaced by muscle. With a cloth tape, take measurements of nine sites on your body. Note all of your results in the AstroFit chart on page 84 at Day 1, Week 4, Week 8, and finally at Week 12.

To ensure accuracy, use the same tape for each measuring session. Apply the tape lightly to the skin. Make sure that it is taut but not tight. Record the circumference to the nearest eighth of an inch.

- *Neck:* Place the tape midway between your head and shoulders.
- *Shoulder:* Measure your shoulders one inch below the top of your torso.
- *Chest:* Place the tape around your body at the nipple line.
- *Waist:* Measure approximately one inch above your navel.
- *Hips:* With your heels together, put the tape around the widest part of your hips.
- *Right thigh:* Put your right leg forward a few inches and measure just below your buttocks.
- *Right calf:* Measure at the widest part of your calf.
- *Right upper arm:* Hold your arm straight out in front of you (palm facing up). Wrap the tape measure at the widest part of your upper arm.
- *Right forearm:* Still holding your arm out in front of you, measure the widest part of your forearm.

4. Have Someone Take Full-Body Photographs of You in a Bathing Suit

Most people have a mental picture of how they look. However, staring at a full-body photo of yourself gives you a very clear idea of where you are and where you want to go. Before you begin your AstroFit Program, have a trusted friend take "before" photographs of you.

- Wear a snug bathing suit. You're looking for contrast, so pose against a light background if you are wearing a dark suit, or a dark background if you are wearing a light suit. Women should wear a two-piece suit so their waistline is clearly visible.
- Use black-and-white film. This will highlight your body and not your clothing and surroundings.
- Stand relaxed and have three photos taken from three different positions: front, right side, and back. For all the photos, place your hands on top of your head. For the back and front poses, keep your heels shoulder width apart. Relax. Do not suck in your belly or flex your muscles.
- Have the film processed and prints made. On the back of each photograph, write the date, your body fat percentage, and your BMI.

Repeat the photo session at the end of Weeks 4, 8, and 12. Be sure to wear the same bathing suit and assume the same poses.

How Fit Are You?

Your current level of physical fitness—how strong you are, what the extent of your aerobic endurance is, and how flexible you are—will give you a good idea of where you currently stand on the aging continuum. The fitter you are, the further back you can turn the clock.

I find that many people have unrealistic notions about their current level of fitness. They think they're stronger and more limber than they actually are. Use the following tests as a starting point in helping personalize your training program. They will provide you with a clear picture of where you are now and point out specific areas that need work.

You can easily perform these tests at home by yourself, although having someone time your efforts will make it much easier. All you need is comfortable workout clothing and a stopwatch (a watch with a secondhand will do).

The first series of tests assess your muscular endurance, the second measures the aerobic endurance of your heart and lungs, and the third evaluates your overall flexibility. Again, if you've been relatively inactive or have high blood pressure, arthritis, diabetes, or any other health problem, be sure to check with your physician before taking these tests.

Muscular Endurance

First measure the overall muscular endurance of your upper, middle, and lower body with the following three basic tests.

Lower-Body Strength

WALL SIT

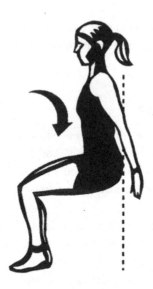

What It Does

This test measures the strength of your thigh (quadriceps) muscles.

How to Do It

1. Stand and lean your back against a wall. Place your feet flat on the floor and shoulder width apart, approximately two feet from the wall.

2. Gently slide down the wall until your upper thighs are at an approximately 45-degree angle to the floor and you are in a "sitting" position.

3. Time yourself as you hold this position for as long as you can without knee discomfort. Record your result on your AstroFit chart on page 84.

Abdominal Strength

ABDOMINAL HOLD

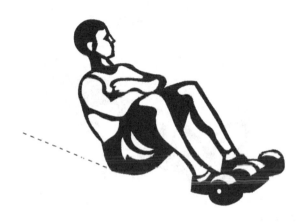

What It Does

This tests the strength of your abdominal muscles, which is critical to good posture and to preventing lower back problems.

How to Do It

1. Lie on your back on the floor with your knees bent at a 45-degree angle. Your feet should be flat on the floor.

2. Cross your hands over your chest and raise your shoulders until they form a 45-degree angle with the floor.

3. Timing yourself, hold this position for as long as you can. Record your results on your AstroFit chart on page 84.

Upper-Body Strength

PUSH-UP

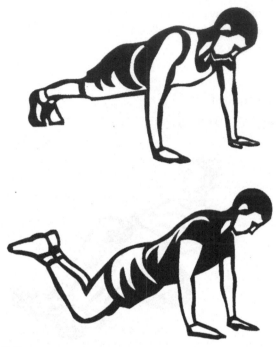

What It Does

Push-ups are an excellent indicator of upper-body muscle strength.

How to Do It

Perform as many classic push-ups as you are able. If it's too hard, perform this modified version:

1. Lie facedown on the floor, your legs together. Keep your hands at the sides of your chest, palms flat on the floor.
2. Straighten your arms, keep your back flat, and, using your knees as the pivot point, push your upper legs and chest off the floor.
3. Lower yourself back down to the floor, touching the floor with your chin. Your chest, abdomen, and thighs should not touch the floor. This counts as one repetition.

4. Repeat as many as you can without pausing while maintaining the proper push-up form. Record your results on your AstroFit chart on page 84.

Your Muscular Endurance Test Results

Check your scores against the chart below to determine your current strength. These scores are for men in their thirties, women's scores will be approximately 20 percent less than for men. On average, scores decrease approximately 15 percent each decade.

Wall Sit	Abdominal Hold	Push-ups
High: 77 seconds	High: 21 seconds	High: 21
Average: 51 seconds	Average: 13 seconds	Average: 13
Low: Less than 26 seconds	Low: Less than 4 seconds	Low: Fewer than 4

Aerobic Endurance

STEP-UP

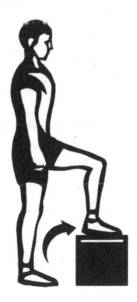

What It Does

The step-up test is a reliable indicator of your current cardiovascular endurance—how well your heart pumps blood through your body—and your general health. In general, a lower exercising heart rate typically indicates a very fit heart muscle. You need a hard surface to step on that is at least eight inches higher than the floor. A staircase step will do.

How to Do It

1. Stand in front of the step. Step up with your right leg, following with your left. Step down on your right leg, following with your left. Each up-up-down-down cycle is one repetition. Aim for 2 repetitions every five seconds.

2. Step up and down for three minutes without stopping, then rest for thirty seconds.

3. Place your index and middle fingers just below the base of your thumb and just above the tendons on your arm. Move your fingertips around until you locate a strong, steady pulse. Count the number of beats in ten seconds. Multiply this number by three to determine beats per thirty seconds. Record your results on your AstroFit chart on page 84.

Your Aerobic Endurance Test Results

Men, check your scores against the chart below to determine your current strength.

NUMBER OF HEARTBEATS			
AGE	30–39	40–49	50+
Excellent	35–38	37–39	37–40
Good	39–41	40–42	41–43
Average	42–43	43–44	44–45
Fair	44–47	45–49	46–49
Poor	48–59	50–60	50–62

Women, compare your results with the following chart.

NUMBER OF HEARTBEATS

AGE	30–39	40–49	50+
Excellent	39–42	41–43	41–44
Good	43–45	44–45	45–47
Average	46–47	46–47	48–49
Fair	48–53	48–54	50–55
Poor	54–66	55–67	56–66

Note: If you become exhausted at any time during the test, do not continue. Score yourself in the poor category, and look forward to improving in the future.

Flexibility

SIT-REACH

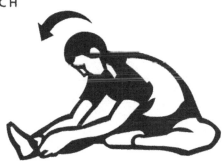

What It Does

This exercise tests the flexibility of your hamstring muscles (located on the backs of your thighs) and is a good indicator of overall muscle flexibility.

How to Do It

1. Sit on the floor. Extend your left leg straight out in front of you. Bend your right leg so that the sole of your right foot touches the inside of your left knee.
2. Gently lean forward at your waist and try to touch your head to your left knee.

Your Flexibility Test Results

If you have good flexibility, you should be able to touch your knee (if you're a woman) or come within two inches of it (if you're a man). Record your results on your AstroFit chart on page 84.

A Baseline to Build On

Once you know your baseline muscular, aerobic, and flexibility levels, you have a foundation on which to build. After the first, second, and third months of your AstroFit program, repeat the tests and chart your progress. You should see improvements in all areas. Remember that a high score in one element of endurance doesn't balance out a poor score in another. Your overall goal is to score well in each test.

Three

Putting the AstroFit Program
into Action

6

Design Your AstroFit Plan

Be of good cheer. Do not think of today's failures, but of the success that may come tomorrow. You have set yourselves a difficult task, but you will succeed if you persevere; and you will find a joy in overcoming obstacles.
—HELEN KELLER

As I sit here writing this, I'm thinking about my father, William T. Evans. Dad was a Marine Corps engineer for three decades and a patriotic, hardworking man who completed two tours of duty in Vietnam while I was growing up. Tragically, he shortchanged himself when it came to his own health. Like many of his contemporaries, my father carried too much weight. He ate the wrong kinds of foods. A lifelong cigarette smoker and infrequent exerciser, Dad was only sixty-nine years old when he died.

I'm certain that if my father had done resistance training and lost the extra pounds, he might have been inspired to eliminate the cigarettes that triggered his emphysema. He might still be here with me, enjoying time with my wife, Betsey, and his three grandchildren, whom he never had a chance to meet. I miss my father every single day, but what makes his loss even harder to accept is knowing that AstroFit would have made a profound difference in his life.

I am committed to avoiding the mistakes that my father made. My personal hope is to become a grandfather to my children's children, the kind of grandfather my children grew up without. I also

hope to serve as a role model for sensible aging so that my children—
and grandchildren—will benefit from the example I set.

How I Start My Day

Just a tick past the half-century mark, I start each workday by kiss-
ing Betsey good-bye as she sets off on her daily six-mile run with our
dog, Grace. Hopping onto my mountain bike, I begin my eleven-mile
ride to work. Most rides generally prove to be an interesting adventure. The trip typically takes forty-five minutes in the morning. The
tough days are when the thermometer hovers around 105° F. and
angry motorists roll down their windows and yell at me to get off the
road. I just put my head down and keep pedaling.

With my muscles completely warmed up after my commute, and
sweating profusely, I then go through my E-Centric weight machine
workout three mornings a week. At my Reynolds Center exercise lab
I have a complete set of Keiser compressed-air weight machines.
Keiser makes a state-of-the-art weight-training setup that allows me
to simply press a button on the machine handle—no weight stacks or
weight selector pins to deal with—and I can increase or decrease the
resistance automatically without stopping the exercise, even if I'm in
the middle of a repetition.

I start my E-Centric workout with bench presses. Getting the
pressure up to 150 pounds, I raise the bar to the count of two, then
slowly lower it back to my chest, mentally counting out six seconds.
I pause briefly and then push the weight up again, repeating the raising and lowering ten times. This is a good starting exercise for me.
My muscles are getting warmed up, and the message is being sent out
to my brain to recruit other muscles for the upcoming workout.

Next on my schedule are biceps curls, so I switch machines. I set
the resistance and begin slowly curling the weight up to my shoulders, then slowly lowering it back down. My arms strain against the
resistance, and it's a good feeling. By the eighth repetition, my arms
are quivering from the effort, but I maintain my strict form and finish to the tenth and last repetition.

After catching my breath, I begin triceps extensions. This exercise builds the muscles at the back of my arms. I set the weight, which is five pounds more than I had been using for almost a month, and prepare myself mentally for the lift. These muscles are my weakness, and I tell myself to remain focused throughout the exercise. It will be a struggle, I know. By the seventh repetition my arms are trembling, and I wonder if I can go on. I take a deep breath, raise the weight, and then slowly let it back down. I finally make it to the tenth repetition. My arms are tired, but I'm elated. In my previous workout I couldn't make it past seven reps. This is definitely progress.

Side arm raises come next, and I suddenly find that I'm moving the weight with a power I didn't know I possessed. Some days, and only with some particular exercises, you will get this fleeting sensation. You feel as if you have the strength of two people and the exercise poses little difficulty. I make a mental note that perhaps I should raise the weight for this exercise by 5 percent for the next workout. It's fine-tuning the routine like this that keeps the exercises fresh and challenging.

My T-shirt is damp at this point. I take in huge gulps of air as I get myself mentally ready for abdominal work. After setting the resistance level, I grab the handles and pull forward, bending at the waist as far as I can. Holding steady against the pressure, I ease myself back to the starting point, counting to six. I feel my abdominal muscles tense against the resistance, and by the tenth repetition perspiration is running off my arms in rivulets.

The back extension exercise is next, and I flash to the time five years previously, when an acute lower back problem had me in agony for more than two weeks. My back hurt so much that I was unable to perform simple tasks such as tying my shoes or bending over to pick up a pencil. The back extension exercise is my insurance policy that this will not happen again. As I knock off each repetition, I can feel the muscles tense and then relax. As I blast through to the tenth repetition, I'm breathing hard again.

It's time for leg work. I move to the next machine and adjust the height and weight so I can begin my heel raises to strengthen my calf muscles. Pushing up against the resistance is the easy part of the ex-

ercise. Going back down is something else altogether. By the last repetition, my calf muscles feel as if they are on fire. Resisting the
weight as I slowly lower my heels to the start is difficult, but this exercise puts me into the mental frame of mind I need to do squats, the
next exercise on the schedule.

The squat has been called the "king of all exercises" because it's
the one strength-training exercise that brings into play so many muscles—leg, butt, lower back, and abdomen. With the bar set at slightly
below shoulder height, I slowly go down, bending my knees and
counting off the seconds, until the tops of my thighs are almost parallel to the floor at the count of six. As I push to complete the last few
reps, I tell myself I'm getting stronger!

I finish off the workout with two additional leg exercises. The knee
extension builds the quadriceps muscles on the front of my thighs.
These muscles are critical for walking up stairs, running, and getting
up from a chair. After I finish with the quads, I begin knee flexion,
which strengthens the hamstring muscles on the back of my thighs.
Since the hamstrings are much weaker than the quads, I use a lower
resistance and then push through the ten repetitions.

Keeping a Training Diary

My E-Centric workout is over for the day, and I congratulate myself.
It was certainly challenging. I'm well into year two on this particular
program, and I've developed a keen sense of time. Even without looking at the clock, I know that it took me less than twenty-five minutes
to perform the entire routine. As I towel off, I record my workout in
my training diary.

Consistency is a key element in your exercise program if you are
going to achieve your goals. A record-keeping system that charts such
daily variables as weight, morning resting heart rate, workout heart
rate, specific exercise routines, and personal thoughts can provide a
handy record of your progress. As you move along, you may find that
you want to experiment with different exercise routines. With a
training diary you'll be able to note the effects of the new program ac-

curately, referring to it whenever you need to study developing patterns.

You can purchase a training diary in most sporting goods stores. Although these diaries are generally meant expressly for runners, bicyclists, and triathletes, you can easily modify them for your own home use and note down all the pertinent information just after finishing your workout. Of course, you can also use a regular memo book, notebook, or ledger. Include:

- Date
- Time of day
- Body weight (optional)
- Time spent warming up and stretching
- Exercises performed
- Amount of weight lifted
- Any difficulties during the workout
- Scale of overall enjoyment

Over time, with enough workouts written in your training diary, you'll become your own coach. From weekly reviews of your training log, you'll soon see that patterns emerge in your workouts. You'll get a true sense of what your body is actually capable of and how you are progressing.

Brenda Starts the AstroFit Program

With determination and consistency, anyone can reach my level of endurance and muscular strength using AstroFit. When I told this to Brenda, she was incredulous. "That's not fair," she said. "I'm sure you were never in the terrible physical condition that I'm in. I haven't done anything in years, unless you count line dancing."

I explained to Brenda that the beauty of the AstroFit program is that each workout prepares and conditions you to move to the next level, building upon a solid strength base. The Level One workouts that I wanted her to perform were progressive—she would do a little

Sample Training Diary

Date/Time: Monday, July 3, 8:30 A.M.
Workout intensity: 10   Workout enjoyment (1–10): 8
Body weight: 195
Warm-up/Stretches: Bicycle, 30 minutes

Exercise	Weight (lbs.)	Sets	Reps
Bench press	150	1	10
Biceps curl	100	1	10
Triceps extension	40	1	10
Side-arm raises	30	1	10
Abdominal curls	130	1	10
Back extension	75	1	10
Calf raise	150	1	10
Squat	350	1	10
Knee extension	100	1	10
Knee flexion	75	1	10

Workout thoughts:

Felt a little tired for the first ten minutes, but that may have been related to the hot temperatures (110° F.) while riding in today. Drink more water! For Wednesday's workout, need to increase weight by five pounds on my side-arm raises. Stay tougher mentally on the knee flexion. Don't forget the afternoon protein shake!

more at each workout—and specifically designed with the deconditioned person in mind.

"You will be able to handle your own body weight in these first stages," I told her, "just as I now handle heavy weights two years into the program. Keep at it, and you have my assurance that over time you will rapidly move through each level of AstroFit, lifting heavier dumbbells as your strength and endurance increase to levels you never dreamed yourself capable of before."

Brenda, a forty-five-year-old working mother of four who had ignored her own physical needs for years, was up for the challenge and decided to change her life the AstroFit way.

I'll never forget her first day in the training area of my laboratory. She was apprehensive and unsure of herself. After a ten-minute warm-up on a stationary bike, she got down on the mat and completed four push-ups. While her goal was to finish ten, four was a great start, I told her. As a rule, women generally do not have strong shoulders and arms, but with regular training they can make truly impressive gains.

I next showed Brenda how to perform the shoulder dips on the edge of the weight bench. This exercise is great for developing the triceps muscles at the back of the upper arm. She smiled when I mentioned that it was the best for getting rid of the "jiggles," the weak, flapping underarms that so many women complain about.

Although Brenda could complete only five of the dip repetitions, slowly lowering herself down in six seconds off the bench and then raising herself back up in two seconds, she said she could feel the muscles being exercised on the back of her arms and that it was a good feeling.

Biceps curls were next on our list. Since Brenda would be controlling the resistance, the key here, I told her, was exerting enough pressure on her exercising arm so that she got a good workout. Grabbing her right wrist with her left hand, she slowly lowered her right arm to waist level, resisting all the while as she applied the pressure with her left hand.

After completing this six-second descent and two-second return to the starting point ten times, she was smiling. "For the first time in my life, I could feel my arm muscles come alive," she said.

Brenda then moved on to working her abdominals with an E-Centric sit-up. Sitting on the mat with her feet flat on the floor, she slowly lowered herself back to the count of six until her body was at a 45-degree angle to the mat. By the seventh repetition, she was struggling to bring herself back to the starting point, but she showed her true fighting spirit and finished off the tenth repetition with a rebel yell. "I did it!" she cried, and then fell back flat on the mat and raised her clenched fists.

Brenda had complained of a chronic soreness in her lower back, due in part to her office job, which kept her at her desk for most of the workday. I told her that she'd get some quick relief from the cobra, the next exercise on the program. Lying face down, with her palms flat on the mat next to her shoulders, she slowly pushed her upper body off the mat by straightening her elbows. By the eighth repetition, Brenda's lower back had loosened up enough that she was finally able to keep her hips on the mat as she stared at the ceiling and tilted her spine back. Standing up, she said that she felt both strengthened and stretched by this particular exercise.

For developing overall strength and balance, there is no better exercise than the squat. Holding on to two towels looped around doorknobs and with her feet positioned shoulder width apart and flat on the mat, Brenda slowly lowered herself down to the count of six until her thighs were almost parallel to the mat. She lost her balance twice as she struggled to raise herself to the upright starting position, but I assured her that as her legs and abdominal muscles became stronger over the next few workout sessions, poor balance would no longer be an issue. When she completed her tenth repetition, she was perspiring lightly.

Lunges, which help strengthen the hips and legs and ensure balance, were the last exercises for Brenda. After showing her the proper form, she had her doubts that she could do all ten lunges because her legs felt like Jell-O. After struggling to complete the ten repetitions, stepping out with her right foot and then slowly lowering her left knee to the mat, she shook her head slowly and then smiled.

Her cheeks were now pink, and her hair was matted with perspiration. "It was tough," she admitted, "but it felt great at the same time. I feel energized. I can do this."

And she has. Brenda is now on to Level Two workouts, using dumbbells for one set of ten repetitions. She has already tripled her strength and lost close to ten pounds. For someone who had serious doubts about her ability to undertake the E-Centric training program, her achievements after sixty days have convinced Brenda that AstroFit can work for anyone.

Getting Started: What You Will Need

WORKOUT AREA

You don't need a lot of space, but don't shortchange yourself. Set aside an area with plenty of room for your equipment. A full-length mirror is a plus because exercising in front of it helps ensure proper form. Finally, a sound system with your favorite CDs or a TV will certainly help bolster your workout enjoyment.

WORKOUT CLOTHING

Invest in clothing that makes you feel athletic. Cotton and breathable synthetics work best because they either absorb or wick away perspiration and keep you cool. Shorts and shirts need to be loose-fitting and comfortable. If your shirt or shorts bind or chafe you, you will have difficulty achieving proper form. Have a good-sized cotton towel handy to wipe the sweat from your brow and equipment.

Sturdy, comfortable shoes that provide good ankle support and have solid arches will help you maintain balance and protect your feet. I don't recommend exercising barefoot. Not only can your feet slip on the rug or floor, but you risk greater injury if you accidentally drop a dumbbell on your foot.

Gloves are not a must, but padded gloves provide a better grip on the dumbbells and reduce the formation of calluses.

WEIGHTS

If and when you are ready to move on to Level Two of the program, you will need some dumbbells to provide resistance. Dumbbells are quite inexpensive—expect to pay between $5 and $20 for a pair of cast-iron weights, depending on the poundage—and can be purchased at any major sporting goods store. In order to best maximize your workouts and make the greatest gains, I suggest that you purchase several pairs of dumbbells of different weights. Since some exercises may be more demanding than others, having the different weights will allow you to use lighter or heavier dumbbells for each one.

Men should consider sets of 8-, 10-, 12-, 15-, 20-, 25-, and possibly 30-pound weights. Women should consider sets of 3-, 5-, 8-, 12-, 15-, and 20-pound dumbbells.

If you're very serious about the program (and I'm sure you are), space-conscious, and strong (or expect to be), I recommend a specific set of dumbbells. I have found the PowerBlock to be the perfect home strength-training unit because of its ease of operation. Just slide the selector pin into the rectangular block and lift out a weight, from five through forty-five pounds.

This ingenious weight system (Intellbell, Inc., 1819 South Cedar Avenue, Owatonna, MN 55060; tel: 800-446-5215) is the equivalent of having sixteen pairs of dumbbells conveniently compressed into two handheld adjustable weight stacks. Offering variety, efficiency, and comfort, the PowerBlock is barely larger than a shoe box.

WEIGHT BENCH

A taut, simulated-leather cover on the bench is best for comfort and long bench life. Good-quality benches, sold at sporting goods stores, start at $100 and go up to $400.

EXERCISE BALL

A safe and effective way to build strength, flexibility, and balance is an oversized air-filled ball (also known as a "stability ball" or "Swiss ball"). Made from durable vinyl, the balls come in different sizes to match body weight and height. Can be used in place of a weight bench.

JUMP ROPE

You can jump rope almost anywhere, anytime, getting a good cardiovascular workout while helping build endurance. Think about rope skipping as your pre-E-Centric warm-up. Cotton ropes are a cheap investment. Get a standard nine-foot length, with handles that fit comfortably in your hands. Those with ball bearings work best because they keep the rope revolving smoothly around the handle.

EXERCISE MAT

A mat is extremely useful for pre- and postworkout stretching as well as for some exercises during the workout. Make sure the padding is

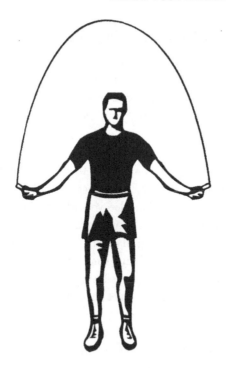

thick enough that your knees and elbows don't push through to the floor.

TRAINING DIARY
Use this to keep track of your exercises, weights, sets, reps, and thoughts on the workouts.

WATER BOTTLE
Drink at least a quart during each workout. You're composed largely of water: approximately 83 percent of your blood is water, 75 percent of your brain is water, and 25 percent of your bones is water. If you lose water in a workout, you have to put it back or you can expect subpar workouts. A loss of 2 to 3 percent of your body weight by sweating can lead to decreased concentration, coordination, strength, and stamina, as well as possible muscle cramps.

The AstroFit Ninety-Day Program

The E-Centric program has been designed to maximize results over a three-month span. All you have to do is follow the instructions for each exercise, and you're guaranteed to see and feel changes. The exercises will work all the basic muscle groups, ensuring balanced strength and stable joints. At the end of three months, you will have succeeded in reversing the "age" of your body!

As part of this program, I want you to do some aerobic exercise on days when you are not doing E-Centrics. Four days of walking, running, swimming, or whatever else you like to do to get your heart pumping will help establish a strong cardiovascular base. I know that if you haven't been exercising in a while, this program may be tiring for you. That's okay. If you find that on Thursday you're still fatigued from E-Centrics on Wednesday and still don't have the energy to go out and walk, feel free to take the extra recovery day.

When you begin your E-Centric training, you will start gaining strength rapidly—even before there is any evidence of muscle growth. Every time you train, your central nervous system becomes more efficient. The impressive gains in strength during the first two months of E-Centrics result from the increased recruitment of existing muscle cells. Even if you're totally out of shape when you start the program, you can expect to regain the muscles of your youth, tripling and even quadrupling your strength in only twelve weeks.

But first, you have to make the commitment to start your ninety-day program. When you do—and I hope you are ready by Monday—you'll soon find that you never felt better or younger. Here's an overview of what's in store for you.

Month 1

Start body-resistance E-Centrics. Also, walk a minimum of every other day for twenty minutes. Try to incorporate more activity into your day. Cut back on fats in your diet, and eat four to six smaller meals a day. Add muscle-building protein to your day with a protein shake after each workout.

Level One E-Centrics: Body-Weight Resistance

Here's something so old—yet effective—that it's new. The Super Seven body-weight exercises in Level One use only the weight of your body as resistance. Exercises such as push-ups, dips, squats, and lunges are well suited to this type of program. Outdated? Perhaps. Underrated? Definitely! These calisthenic—from the Greek *kalos sthenos,* meaning "beautiful strength"—exercises are the perfect way to begin the program: they build muscle and strength by challenging you to take control of your own body weight. A built-in advantage of these low-tech exercises is that you can perform them just about anywhere you want, without the need for any equipment. The AstroFit exercises incorporate basic movements designed to work the major muscle groups, all on the same day.

You probably remember most of these body-weight exercises from gym class. They may be a bit tougher for you now, but they are still effective. Done correctly, the exercises burn calories and body fat while building muscle, endurance, and overall strength.

The aim here is not to see how many repetitions of the exercises you can do but to perform each one flawlessly, session after session. I am asking you to do ten repetitions of each exercise, three days a week. The days off between the workouts are the time to get in your aerobic exercise, such as walking or swimming.

Your focus should be not on how you *look* but on how you *feel.* You will probably experience some soreness for the first week or so, but that's normal. Your muscles are waking up as you reintroduce them to what they were made to do: help you move. Warming up properly (you should break into a light sweat) and cooling down sufficiently (with at least five minutes of walking, swimming, or biking) will help minimize muscle soreness. So will using correct form. Never bounce or jerk your muscles in any exercise movement. This can easily tear muscles or unnaturally push them past their normal length, resulting in injury.

Month 1: Level One E-Centrics
Body-Weight-Resistance Exercises

Follow this workout for the first month, in the order listed.

EXERCISE	SETS/REPS
1. Push-up (p. 120)	1/10
2. Chair dip (p. 122)	1/10
3. Biceps curl (p. 124)	1/10
4. Sit-up (p. 125)	1/10
5. Cobra (p. 126)	1/10
6. Door squat (p. 128)	1/10
7. Forward lunge (p. 129)	1/10

Week 1 Game Plan

Getting started with the program may be the toughest part for you. The best way to do it is to have your workout time set as if you had made an appointment for yourself. By developing this positive, simple habit you will prepare the way for a profound lifetime improvement.

Before you begin, take all your vital measurements (body fat percentage, body mass index, weight, and nine circumference checkpoints) and record them on your AstroFit chart on page 84. Keep this chart handy, as you will be returning to it each month. You can also record your numbers in your training diary. Have someone take your "before" photographs.

Get in your twenty minutes of cardiovascular work, either walking, swimming, or bicycling. Aim for every other day. Try daily if you already have a high level of fitness. Don't forget to drink plenty of fluids—at least one quart daily of water or fruit juice. You're exercising and need to replace what is lost through perspiration. You'll know you're drinking enough if you have to go to the bathroom between four and eight times daily.

Learn each exercise and practice performing it correctly. When you exercise with correct form, you train your muscles to support your body throughout the day. Perfect form will become even more important when you add weights to your workout in a month.

Week 2 Game Plan

If you weren't able to complete the full number of repetitions in some of the exercises last week, aim to go for the complete ten this week. Keep up your aerobic exercise; you may notice that it seems slightly easier. To avoid boredom, consider walking in the opposite direction. Note all of your thoughts in your training diary. Be sure to get in your daily protein. Your choices include soy, egg whites, whey powder, tofu, chicken, fish, beans, tuna, cottage cheese, and beef.

Week 3 Game Plan

Review the major workout goals you want to achieve for the upcoming week. Some of the E-Centrics may be easier to perform now. If you find that they are not as challenging as you would like, don't add weight, add repetitions. Drink a protein shake after each workout. If you have to travel for business this week, get up early and perform the workout before your first meeting. You'll feel energized and alert. If you haven't missed a single workout yet, reward yourself.

You have a "vital statistics day" coming up next week. Consider buying a bioimpedence scale to measure your fat percentage. Remember, fat loss is what matters most in this program.

Week 4 Game Plan

Try waking up forty-five minutes earlier than usual and getting in your workout first thing after you get up. For those of you who have already made tremendous progress with E-Centrics, increase your repetitions to the twelve- to fifteen-rep range for each exercise. This week, try to add five to ten more minutes to your regular cardiovascular activities. If that's not possible, aim for an additional daily session. Consider an early-evening walk with a loved one.

At the end of the week, take all of your vital measurements again and record them on your AstroFit chart on page 84. Enlist your photographer to take your photographs again, wearing the same bathing suit.

Congratulations! You have completed thirty days of age-reversing, fat-burning, muscle-building E-Centric exercise!

Month 2

This month you begin pumping iron. The exercises work the same muscles that you exercised the previous month, but dumbbells will be providing the resistance. You want to see strength increases, and you will. Continue your cardiovascular workouts. Why not try something different this month, such as swimming or an aerobics class?

Level Two E-Centrics: With Dumbbells

The eight exercises in Level Two use dumbbells for resistance and introduce your muscles to the challenge of free weights. Your goal is to exercise your muscles to the level of fatigue by the tenth repetition. Before lifting any weight, familiarize yourself with each exercise. Carefully study the descriptions and illustrations. If something looks difficult or you're unsure, seek out someone with more experience who is willing to help. A couple of sessions with a certified personal trainer are a good investment.

Your goal is not to see how much weight you can lift but rather to increase muscle mass and enhance strength. Use very light dumbbells. I don't want you to be working anywhere close to your maximum strength.

Week 5 Game Plan

You're progressing, but there's a lot more to be done this month. Begin by determining how much weight you will lift for each exercise. This may take some guesswork, so leave yourself some extra time in the first two workouts to find the weight you can lift with

Month 2: Level Two E-Centrics
Weight-Resistance Exercises

Follow this workout for the second month, in the order listed.

EXERCISE	SETS/REPS
1. Biceps curl with dumbbell (p. 133)	1/10
2. Dumbbell chest press (p. 134)	1/10
3. Side-arm raise with dumbbells (p. 136)	1/10
4. Abdominal curl with dumbbell (p. 137)	1/10
5. Cobra (p. 138)	1/10
6. Standing heel raise with dumbbell (p. 140)	1/10
7. Squat with dumbbells (p. 141)	1/10
8. Forward lunge with dumbbells (p. 143)	1/10

good form for ten repetitions. If you find that you can do more than ten and don't feel daunted by the weight, it's too light. Try a 5 percent increase and see how you manage.

Continue with your aerobic workouts for a minimum of twenty minutes every other day. If you can do more, it shows you're making real progress. If you're using soy as your protein supplement, consider a switch to whey protein this week and see how you like it.

Week 6 Game Plan

Before each workout, sit alone for five minutes and review your goals for the session. You should have your weights down for all of your exercises by now. Concentrate on proper form. If you have to increase the weight for one exercise, do so, but don't move up for all of them. You'll find that you make progress rapidly in some exercises, while others will take a little longer. Two up, six down. If you can't keep that cadence while maintaining good form, reduce the weight. If you feel tired after a hard workout, don't worry. You've worked your muscles, and they're recovering. Take a nap, if you can, and you'll awaken refreshed.

Week 7 Game Plan

Evaluate your progress by how vital and energetic you now feel, not just by how much weight you are lifting. Pencil at least an hour of relaxation time into your schedule this week. Instead of eating the "old way"—three big meals, with the biggest in the evening—make a concerted effort to switch to the "new way" and consume four to six minimeals every day. With your stronger leg muscles, always take the stairs instead of the elevator. You have your next day of reckoning coming up next week!

Week 8 Game Plan

Continue with the same weights as last week. If you haven't added any weight in two weeks, consider going up 5 percent in those exercises that don't seem as taxing. Accept the challenge. Even though you have eliminated many old favorites from your diet, you can enjoy a slice of pizza once in a while. Your motto should be "everything in moderation." Keep up your cardiovascular activities. If you're a golfer, leave the cart and walk the eighteen holes. You're much fitter now than you realize.

At the end of Week 8, take all of your vital measurements again and record them on your AstroFit chart on page 84. Enlist your photographer to take your photographs again, wearing the same bathing suit.

Congratulations! You have completed sixty days of age-reversing, fat-burning, muscle-building E-Centric exercise!

Month 3

Four more weeks to go. Your technique is now solid, and your muscles are primed for growth and fat burning.

Level Three E-Centrics: Accept the Challenge

The exercises this month stay the same, but you'll add more repetitions and/or more weight. Pick a day when you're well rested and really go at the weights. Push for twelve to fifteen reps of a challenging exercise, or increase the weight by ten pounds and go for five reps. Or try to finish off two sets of the entire routine. This may just be what it takes to help you break through to a new level of strength—and give yourself a boost of self-confidence as well.

Check the short-term goals you wrote down two months ago. How many have you achieved so far? Take time out to plan how you can achieve them all. Write down your strategies in your diary.

Week 9 Game Plan

Try to get in five twenty-minute sessions of aerobic exercise this week. Keep up the E-Centric cadence: two up, six down. Make a list in your training diary of five goals you want to achieve this week. It's very satisfying to check each one off as you meet or exceed the goal.

Week 10 Game Plan

Great form is more important than heavy weights. Resist the urge to increase the weight unless you really can manage to keep the E-Centric cadence for the full ten reps without cheating. Now that you're doing so well, think about teaching a beginner what has taken you so long to learn.

Week 11 Game Plan

Two more weeks to go. Try adding 5 percent to most exercises if you haven't already. Aerobics are key. How about dancing sometime this week? It's great exercise and lots of fun. You'll probably need new clothes, since your old ones are most likely too baggy.

Week 12 Game Plan

Three more E-Centric sessions left. Don't aim for big breakthroughs this week. Success comes in small steps, not huge leaps. Come to the realization that these past three months have been a celebration of good health and a happy life.

One more measuring session. Compare your statistics against those from Day 1. Amazing, right? If your bathing suit is too loose for the photo session, tighten it in the back.

E-Centrics for the Future

Congratulations! You have now laid the foundation for a strong, shapely physique. Continue performing one or two sets of each exercise; the choice is yours. If you try two sets, for the first set of every movement, use as heavy a weight as you can handle for six reps. Then, after a short rest, reduce the weight to permit you to perform a second set of ten repetitions.

You will have to experiment to determine how much weight you can use in the first set and how much you will have to reduce it for the second. In some exercises, it may be only a few pounds. In others it may entail a reduction of as much as 25 percent of the weight of the previous set. Once again, trial and error is the best method for determining the weight. Alternating high-weight and low-weight reps like this allows you to add variety to the program, and using heavier weights will increase your muscle strength dramatically and develop additional endurance.

On the Value of Persistence

When it comes to age reversal, too many people are looking for a quick fix—a pill or potion that will keep you younger, melt away fat, increase lean muscle, and make you run faster and jump higher. I have a secret for you: it doesn't exist. Physical change is hard earned and will come only through the accumulation of hundreds of hours of work put in on a daily basis. To keep you from feeling overwhelmed, I want you to focus on taking one workout, one day at a time. Granted, there will be times when you feel that you're not making progress and you may even question why you're exercising. Take solace in knowing that you're not alone.

I penciled this quote from Jacob Riis into my workout log many years ago, and it helps me put exercise and so many other things into perspective. Riis, who lived from 1849 to 1914, was a prominent New York social reformer, news reporter, and photographer. I refer to this quotation often because I think it succinctly sums up the value of daily effort and persistence, not only in keeping to your exercise goals but in helping achieve your life dreams as well:

When nothing seems to help, I go and look at the stonecutter hammering away at his rock, perhaps a hundred times without as much as a crack showing in it. Yet, at the hundred and first blow, it will split in two; and I know it was not that blow that did it, but all that had gone before.

7

Level One E-Centrics: The Super Seven

What we hope ever to do with ease, we must learn first to do with diligence.
—SAMUEL JOHNSON

The Level One workout is the beginning of a twelve-week, triple-phase muscle-building program designed to take you from a very low level of overall fitness to a much higher one. The advantage of the Super Seven exercises is that while they are deceptively simple and require little or no equipment—two towels and a sturdy chair are all you need—they still offer effective ways of challenging your muscles with body-weight resistance. It's just you against gravity. Your muscles don't know the difference between dumbbells, gym equipment, and your own body weight; they respond to anything that offers resistance. *You are the weight in this instance.*

By raising and slowly lowering your arms, legs, or torso, by changing the angle of your body position, or by shifting your center of gravity, you will begin to build muscle. And you'll do it without lifting dumbbells or using typical strength-training equipment found in the gym.

To ensure the best workout possible, follow these guidelines:

- *Forget about time.* Each workout should take about twenty to thirty minutes. Don't be concerned about the time, however. I want you to focus on perfect form while performing each exercise.

- *Warm up before you begin.* In order to prepare the body for the stress of exercise, begin each workout with a warm-up program of two to five minutes. By warming up before you exercise—jumping rope, running in place, riding a stationary bike—you will gradually raise your body temperature, increase blood flow to the muscles, accelerate your heart rate, gently stretch your muscles, and prepare all your body joints for exercise. You will know you're ready to start your workout session when you begin to perspire. Complete your warm-up with some gentle stretching.

- *Maintain proper form.* Follow the recommended form for each exercise. Incorrect form can reduce the load on the muscle group that you want to develop, or, more important, lead to injury by overstressing joints and tendons.

- *If possible, perform the exercises in front of a full-length mirror.* Play close attention to the line your torso makes, the positioning of your arms, and the angle of your legs in the various exercises.

- *Perform each repetition the E-Centric way.* Two seconds up, six seconds down. Move your body smoothly through your full range of motion. The more slowly you are able to lower your body, the more you will overload, and therefore develop, your muscles.

- *Cool down when you're finished.* Cooling down after a workout is just as important as warming up. This will prevent "pooling" of the blood in the large arteries of the legs. Coming to a sudden stop can trigger a quick drop in blood pressure. In some cases, this can cause light-headedness or dizziness.

  Your aim is to gradually return your cardiovascular system to almost a preworkout condition with five minutes of slow stretching or aerobics. Cooling down adequately can also reduce muscle stiffness. Lactic acid, a natural waste product produced by the muscles during exercise, builds up during the latter stages of exercise and may cause the muscles to ache. The accumulation of lactic acid is a normal and temporary condition that can be greatly alleviated by a cool-down period.

- *Work your way up to ten repetitions.* Performing one set of each exercise is enough to develop metabolically active lean muscle mass. Moreover, this is a relatively quick program you can perform anywhere, which is especially convenient when you're just beginning to work E-Centric training into your life and schedule.

Five Rules to Remember

When performing the Super Seven:

- *Keep your body in one plane.* Do not bend forward at the hip or arch your back.
- *Focus your gaze* on a particular point at about eye level.
- *Keep breathing normally* as you exercise. Exhale during the most difficult part of the exercise. Inhale during the easiest part of the exercise.
- *Perform each exercise ten times* (ten repetitions). Rest for one to two minutes before beginning the next exercise.
- *Perform this program three times a week.*

Level One E-Centric Exercises

1. Push-up—modified or classic (shoulders, back, neck)
2. Chair dip (shoulders, arms, back)
3. Biceps curl (arms)
4. Sit-up (abdomen)
5. Cobra (back, hips, neck)
6. Door squat (back, hips, knees)
7. Forward lunge (back, hips, knees)

EXERCISE 1: MODIFIED PUSH-UP

This exercise can quickly strengthen your shoulders, arms, and chest. Using only your body weight, you challenge your front deltoids, pectorals, and triceps. In addition, push-ups work your ab-

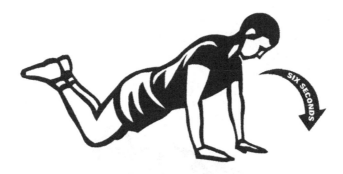

dominal and back muscles. You may find that even your legs and buttocks get a workout. Performing push-ups regularly will give you more than just an aesthetic advantage: the muscles that develop from this exercise can give you the strength needed in any activity requiring arm or chest strength.

You may find that the push-up is not easy to perform. Don't give up! Many women cannot initially perform one full push-up, and men who are generally strong but who do not exercise their upper bodies regularly may also have some difficulty. Keep at it. If five are all you can do, aim for six at your next workout. Before long, you'll be performing ten with ease.

Get Set

- Get down on all fours on an exercise mat or rug with your arms extended, palms flat on the floor, shoulder width apart, fingers pointing forward. Your knees should be bent at slightly more than a 90-degree angle.
- Keep your feet perpendicular to the floor. They can also be up in the air, but do not cross them or you will put extra pressure on your lower back.

E-Centric Phase

- 1-2-3-4-5-6-down. Slowly lower yourself to the floor, touching the floor with your chest.
- Pause for a second.

Upward Movement

- 1-2-up. Keep your back flat, and, using your knees as the pivot point, push your torso away from the floor as you straighten your arms and rise back to the starting position.

Pointer
- Lower and lift your body as a single unit. Don't bend or let your abdomen sag.

EXERCISE 1: CLASSIC PUSH-UP

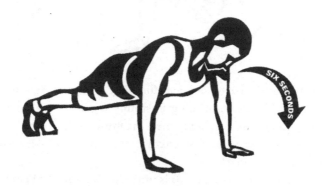

If you've built up enough strength and find the modified push-up to be too easy, perform this classic military version instead.

Get Set
- Lie facedown on the floor with your legs together.
- Keep your hands at the sides of your chest, palms flat on the floor.
- Raise your body onto your hands and toes with your hands now perpendicular to your shoulders.

E-Centric Phase
- 1-2-3-4-5-6-down. Inhale and bend your elbows as you slowly lower your body to within three inches of the floor.
- Pause for one second.

Upward Movement
- 1-2-up. Push back up to the starting position and repeat.

Pointers
- Keep your descents slow, with your back flat.
- Don't continue if you feel any pain or strain in your lower back.

EXERCISE 2: CHAIR DIP

This exercise zeroes in on the triceps muscles on the back of your arms and also exercises the muscles of your shoulders, chest, and

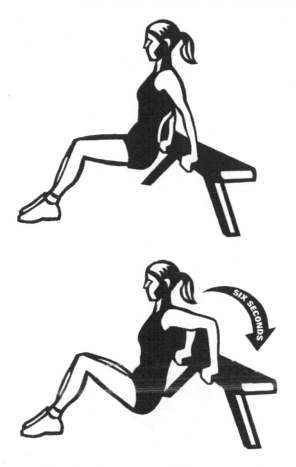

back: the rear deltoids, lower pectorals, lower trapezius, and latissimus.

Get Set

- Sit on the edge of a sturdy chair (to make sure that it doesn't slide, set it against a wall) or weight bench with your hands under your buttocks.
- Keep your hands firmly on the seat.
- Straighten your arms and carefully slide your feet out until your buttocks are off the chair and your legs are straight out in front of you, feet flat on the floor.
- Your arms should be straight.

E-Centric Phase
- 1-2-3-4-5-6-down. Slowly lower yourself down off the chair until your upper arms are parallel to the floor.
- Pause for one second.

Upward Movement
- 1-2-up. Push yourself back up slowly until your arms are straight again and repeat.

Pointers
- Look straight ahead as you dip downward.
- Don't arch your back.
- As you lower yourself, keep your hips and back as close to the chair as possible.
- Stop when your upper arms are parallel to the floor. Going any lower could cause elbow discomfort.

EXERCISE 3: BICEPS CURL

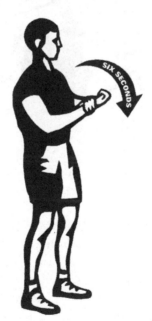

When someone asks you to make a muscle, you immediately flex your biceps. The self-resistance biceps curl strengthens your biceps, the muscles on the front of your upper arm that help you bend your arm. To perform this exercise correctly, you must supply the resistance by tensing your muscles while you perform the downward movement.

Get Set

- Start by standing with your right arm flexed at your side, with your fist closed, fingers in front of your shoulder, as if you were holding a dumbbell.
- Hold the front of your right wrist with your left hand and apply just enough pressure so that it's difficult (but not impossible) to bend your arm.

E-Centric Phase

- 1-2-3-4-5-6-down. Curl your right arm down slowly, fighting the pushing motion of your left hand—thereby creating an E-Centric movement—until your right forearm is parallel to the floor.
- Pause for a second.

Upward Movement

- 1-2-up. Slowly return to the starting position.
- Repeat ten times with your right arm, then switch to your left and repeat.

Pointers

- Keep the resistance steady so you can lower your arm with control.
- Keep your elbows close to your body in both the downward and upward phases.
- Maintain an erect posture as you perform the exercise.

EXERCISE 4: SIT-UP

The E-Centric sit-up is the ultimate exercise to strengthen the upper and lower abdominal muscles.

Get Set

- Sit on the floor with your knees bent and feet flat on the floor, shoulder width apart. Place your feet under a sturdy couch to stabilize your lower body or have someone hold your ankles.
- Cross your arms in front of your chest.
- Tilt your upper body back slightly so it's at less than a 90-degree angle to the floor.

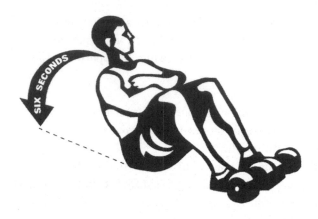

E-Centric Phase

- 1-2-3-4-5-6-down. Slowly lower your upper body toward the floor, curling your torso forward and rounding your lower back, keeping your abdominal muscles contracted.
- When your body reaches a 45-degree angle to the floor, pause for a second.

Upward Movement

- 1-2-up. Slowly rise up to the starting position and repeat.

Pointers

- Lower your body with control.
- Do not hold your breath.
- Do not lower your body lower than a 45-degree angle to the floor. This will shift the stress from your abdominal muscles to your hip flexors or lower back.

EXERCISE 5: COBRA

Our hip flexor muscles tend to tighten as a result of sitting for long periods, and as we age this shortening process contributes to the slumping posture seen in many adults. This classic yoga exercise elongates the hip flexor muscles, reducing pressure and tension on the lower back. The cobra is the best stretching/strengthening exercise for the lower back because it relaxes the back muscles as it gently stretches the muscles of the abdomen, hips, and neck. Since this exercise is designed to stretch *and* strengthen, you will spend an additional few seconds in the upward movement.

Get Set

- Lie on your stomach with your face almost touching the mat.
- Place your palms on the mat at the sides of your shoulders.
- Keep your legs together and the tops of your feet resting on the mat.

Upward Movement

- 1-2-3-4-up. (This exercise has a longer upward phase.) Push up, bringing your head up off the mat.
- Keep your pelvis pushed into the mat while relaxing your buttocks as best you can.
- Slowly arch your spine backward, straightening your elbows.
- Bring your head back and look at the ceiling.
- Pause for a second.

E-Centric Phase

- 1-2-3-4-5-6-down. Descend slowly to the mat, then repeat.

Pointers

- Keep your back relaxed.
- Let your arms do the work as you rise up and descend back to the mat. Don't hunch your shoulders together.
- If your lower back is very stiff, you will not be able to keep your pelvis on the mat. In that case, simply raise your pelvis off the mat as you straighten your arms. As your flexibility increases, you will be able to keep your pelvis on the mat.
- If you're unable to lift up and straighten your arms, begin the exercise propped up on your elbows.

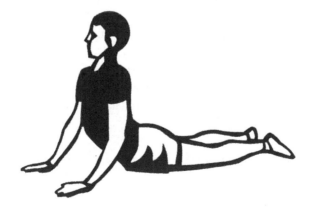

EXERCISE 6: DOOR SQUAT

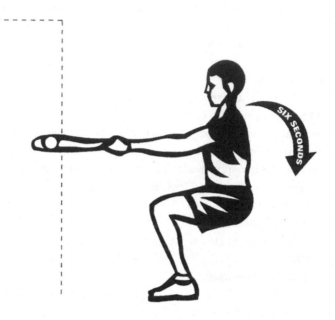

The door squat will strengthen your buttocks, hamstrings, and quadriceps.

Get Set

- Open a sturdy wooden door and loop a bath towel around each doorknob.
- Hold the ends of both towels in your hands. Stand with your arms fully extended in front of you and your feet shoulder width apart.
- Keep your back straight and your weight firmly over your heels.

E-Centric Phase

- 1-2-3-4-5-6-down. Holding on to the towels for balance, slowly squat down as if you were going to sit in a chair, lowering yourself until the tops of your thighs are parallel to the floor.
- Pause for a second.

Upward Movement

- 1-2-up. Pulling on the towels for leverage, slowly rise to the standing position and repeat.

Pointers

- Don't arch your back.
- Concentrate on looking straight ahead.
- As you descend, make sure that your knees travel in the same straight direction that your toes are pointed.
- To ensure knee safety, as you are descending do not let your knees go out farther than your toes.

EXERCISE 7: FORWARD LUNGE

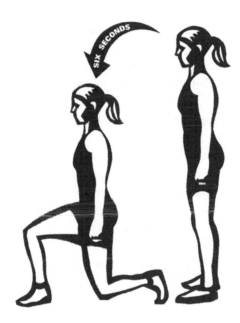

The forward lunge enhances hip flexibility and builds strength in the upper and inner thigh muscles, buttocks, quadriceps, hamstrings, and calves.

Get Set

- Stand with your feet flat on the floor, shoulder width apart.
- Keep your back straight and your hands alongside your hips.
- Slowly take an exaggerated step forward with your right foot as far as possible, keeping your back straight, chest high, chin up, eyes looking forward.

E-Centric Phase

- 1-2-3-4-5-6-down. Slowly bend your right knee to a 90-degree angle, your thigh almost parallel with the floor.
- Lower your left knee until it is a few inches from the ground. Do not let your left knee touch the floor. Your left heel will rise off the floor.
- Balance your weight on your right heel and the toes of your left foot.
- Pause for a second.

Upward Movement

- 1-2-up. Slowly step back to the starting position by straightening your right leg, pushing off from the ball of your foot.
- Step forward with your left foot.
- Complete ten repetitions for each leg.

Pointers

- To maintain proper balance, step straight forward, with your feet shoulder-width apart.
- Don't look down, or you may lose your balance.
- Don't shift your weight forward. Be sure to keep the weight centered directly over your hips to prevent excess pressure on your knees.
- Don't let your knees roll inward or bow outward. This will overstress your knees.
- Don't round your back. This may overstress your lower back.

Don't Forget Your Aerobic Exercise

On your "off" days, I want you to do some form of aerobic activity for twenty minutes or more. This cardiovascular exercise can include brisk walking, jogging, swimming, water aerobics, or the use of various stationary exercise equipment, such as a rower, treadmill, stair climber, or bike. As you become stronger and fitter in the ensuing weeks, I want you to up the ante and perform some aerobic exercise at least six days a week. Believe me, once you get the "exercise bug," you'll be wanting to do more.

8

Level Two E-Centrics: With Dumbbells

Lack of activity destroys the good condition of every human being, while movement and methodical exercise save it and preserve it.
—PLATO

Welcome to the E-Centric workouts with dumbbells. While the body-weight-resistance exercises you completed over the past month have given you a high level of strength and balance, E-Centrics with weights take you even further on the strength continuum. For the next eight weeks you will hoist dumbbells three times a week, performing eight exercises at each session. By the end of each session you will have gone through a full-body workout. Keep the good habits you established in Month 1, such as working on perfect form, adding aerobic exercise to your week, and taking time to warm up and cool down at each workout.

E-Centric Exercises with Dumbbells

The eight exercises in Level Two E-Centrics will eventually become the basis of your Level Three workout. At this stage, light weights will be challenging enough. Later you will be adding heavier weights to challenge your stronger physique.

When it comes to successful training sessions, it's not *how much* you train but *how well* you train. Deviating from the proper form reduces the challenge on the muscle group that you want to develop and, more important, can lead to injury by overstressing joints and tendons. Poor form typically comes from trying to lift too much weight or from lifting heavy weight when you are too tired to lift properly. To make safe but steady progress, err on the lighter side with your dumbbells. Following are some essential points for working out with dumbbells.

Four Rules to Remember

When performing E-Centrics with dumbbells:

- *Pick a weight you can lift at least ten consecutive times, but no more than twelve times.* The last few repetitions should be hard to perform. When you can do twelve repetitions at that weight for two sessions in a row, increase the weight just enough that you can handle ten repetitions at the new weight. Over time you will make big gains by making small, gradual increases in weight.
- *Lift weights in a slow, controlled fashion.* Take two seconds to raise the weights and six seconds to complete the E-Centric lowering phase. Don't hold your breath. Inhale at the beginning of the lift and slowly exhale when you finish the repetition.
- *Perform your E-Centric training three times a week with one rest day in between.* This will allow for adequate muscle recovery and growth.
- *Have fun!* Don't lose your focus on why you are training: to attain personal achievements beyond your exercise goals. See your workout program for what it is: a celebration of life and health.

Level Two E-Centric Exercises with Dumbbells

1. Biceps curl with dumbbells (shoulders, back, neck)
2. Dumbbell chest press (chest, shoulders, arms)

3. Side-arm raise with dumbbells (shoulders, back)
4. Abdominal curl with dumbbells (abdomen)
5. Cobra (back, hips, neck)
6. Standing heel raise with dumbbells (knees, feet, calves)
7. Squat with dumbbells (back, hips, knees, thighs, buttocks, abdomen)
8. Forward lunge with dumbbells (back, hips, knees, thighs, abdomen, buttocks)

EXERCISE 1: BICEPS CURL WITH DUMBBELLS

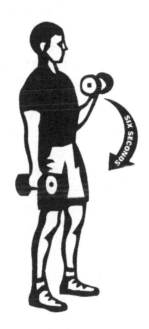

This exercise strengthens the biceps, the two-part muscle involved in lifting and lowering most objects, from small children, luggage, and chairs to bags of groceries and the turkey for your Thanksgiving dinner.

Get Set

- Stand with your back straight and your feet shoulder width apart, holding a dumbbell in each hand at your sides with your palms facing forward.

Upward Movement

- 1-2-up. Lift the left dumbbell up until it touches the front of your shoulders.
- Pause for a second.

E-Centric Phase

- 1-2-3-4-5-6-down. Slowly lower your left arm to the starting position in front of your thighs.
- Repeat the exercise with your right arm.

Pointers

- To maintain the emphasis on the biceps, be sure to keep your elbows firmly in place against your sides as you lift and lower.
- Maintain perfect posture. Do not bend at your waist or swing your elbows out to help raise the weights.
- Lift but don't twist. If you can't lift the weight for each repetition without doing some kind of gyration, reduce the weight and repeat.
- Always look straight ahead as you curl. When you look down, your shoulders automatically hunch forward, making the curl less effective.

EXERCISE 2: DUMBBELL CHEST PRESS

The dumbbell chest press is one of the most popular upper-body exercises. It firms and strengthens your chest, shoulders, and triceps (the backs of your arms).

Get Set

- Sit upright on the floor, a flat weight bench, or a Swiss ball with two dumbbells resting on your thighs. Keep your knees bent and your feet flat on the floor.
- Roll back onto your back and simultaneously bring the dumbbells to the sides of your chest.
- Keep your hands, wrists, and elbows close to your sides.

Upward Movement

- 1-2-up. Slowly straighten your arms and extend the dumbbells directly above your shoulders, with your palms facing forward.

E-Centric Phase

- 1-2-3-4-5-6-down. Slowly bring the dumbbells down to your chest until your elbows are slightly below your torso.

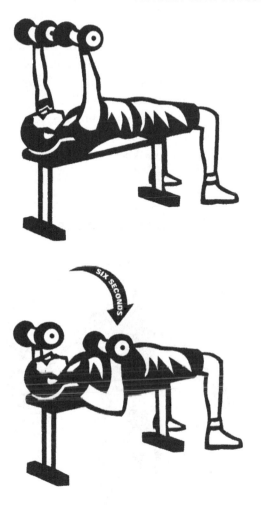

- Stop when your arms form a 90-degree angle, upper arms in line with your shoulders.
- Press the dumbbells back up and repeat.
  Pointers
- To maintain consistency, focus on a spot on the ceiling directly above your chest and press the dumbbells to that point for each repetition.
- Don't lower your elbows deeper than parallel to the floor, or you risk excessive shoulder stress.

- Don't arch your back as you raise or lower the dumbbells or you may injure your spine. If the weights are too heavy to maintain proper form on each repetition, reduce the weights.
- Make sure your wrists are in line with your forearms and elbows. Do not bend your wrists backward.
- To perform this exercise on the floor or an exercise mat, prop several pillows under your shoulder and neck to keep your back slightly elevated. Bend your knees and keep your feet flat on the floor.

EXERCISE 3:
SIDE-ARM RAISE WITH DUMBBELLS

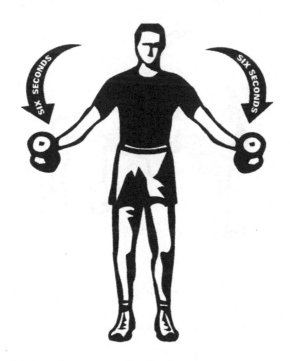

The side-arm raise strengthens the deltoid muscles of your shoulders, which help you raise your arms. Virtually any movement of the arms requires deltoid involvement. While the biceps and triceps flex and extend the elbow joint, it's the deltoids that move the arm around the shoulder joint.

Get Set
- Stand with a dumbbell in each hand.
- Keep your feet flat on the floor, shoulder width apart.
- Bend your knees slightly.
- Hold dumbbells straight down at your sides, with your palms facing inward.

Upward Movement
- 1-2-up. Keeping your shoulders down, lift each of your arms straight out to the sides until the dumbbells are parallel to the ground, as close to shoulder height as possible.
- Hold this position for one second.

E-Centric Phase
- 1-2-3-4-5-6-down. Slowly return to the starting position.
- Repeat the exercise.

Pointers
- Don't lean forward or rock your hips as you raise the dumbbells.
- Don't raise your upper arms higher than parallel to the floor.
- Always stand erect and look straight ahead as you perform each repetition. When you look down, your shoulders automatically hunch forward, making the exercise less effective.

EXERCISE 4:
ABDOMINAL CURL WITH DUMBBELL

This abdominal curl with its E-Centric accent is the ultimate exercise to strengthen the upper and lower abdominal muscles.

Get Set
- Sit on the floor with your knees bent and feet flat on the floor, shoulder width apart. Place your feet under a sturdy couch to stabilize your lower body or have someone hold your ankles.
- Hold one dumbbell in your hand and place both hands on your upper chest.
- Tilt your upper body back so it's less than a 90-degree angle to the floor.

E-Centric Phase
- 1-2-3-4-5-6-down. Slowly lower your upper body toward the floor, curling your torso forward and rounding your lower back, keeping your abdominal muscles contracted.

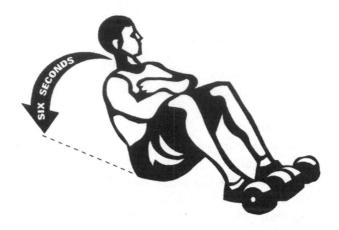

- When your body reaches a 45-degree angle to the floor, pause for a second.
  Upward Movement
- 1-2-up. Slowly rise to the starting position and repeat.
  Pointers
- Lower your body with control.
- Do not hold your breath.
- Do not lower your body below a 45-degree angle to the floor. This will shift the stress from your abdominal muscles to your hip flexors or lower back.

EXERCISE 5: COBRA

In this classic yoga exercise, your spine will slowly undulate like a cobra. Although you don't use any dumbbells when performing this exercise, I've included the cobra because it helps to gently stretch and strengthen the muscles of your lower back and hips, as well as your upper arms. After having done four weeks of cobras in the body-resistance phase, you should now be able to keep your pelvis flat on the mat.

Get Set

- Lie on your stomach with your face almost touching the mat.
- Place your palms on the mat at the sides of your shoulders.
- Keep your legs together and the tops of your feet resting on the mat.

Upward Movement

- 1-2-3-4-up. (This exercise has a longer upward phase.) Push up, bringing your head up off the mat.
- Keep your pelvis pushed into the mat while relaxing your buttocks as best you can.
- Slowly arch your spine backward, straightening your elbows.
- Bring your head back and look at the ceiling.
- Pause for a second.

E-Centric Phase

- 1-2-3-4-5-6-down. Descend slowly to the mat, then repeat.

Pointers

- Keep your back relaxed.
- Let your arms do the work as you rise up and descend back to the mat. Don't hunch your shoulders together.
- If your lower back is very stiff, you will not be able to keep your pelvis on the mat. In that case, simply raise your pelvis off the mat as you straighten your arms. As your flexibility increases, you will be able to keep your pelvis on the mat.

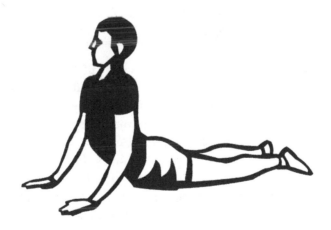

EXERCISE 6:
STANDING HEEL RAISE WITH DUMBBELL

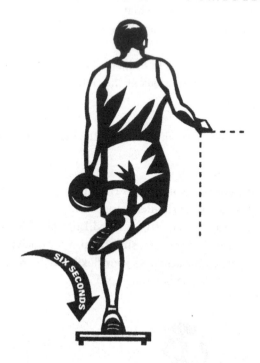

The heel raise strengthens your ankle and calf muscles. All of the leg muscles are used during the complicated muscular task of walking and running, but it's the calf muscles that move the foot and produce the force against the ground that moves you forward. The gastrocnemius is the large diamond-shaped portion of the calf muscle and consists of both fast- and slow-twitch muscle fibers. The other major calf muscle, the soleus, which lies directly beneath the gastrocnemius, is made up almost entirely of fatigue-resistant slow-twitch fibers. The heel raise works both of these muscle fibers maximally.

Get Set

- Holding a dumbbell in your left hand while holding on to a support with your right, stand tall with the ball of your left foot on the edge of a step.
- Put your right foot behind your left leg.

Upward Movement

- 1-2-up. Rise up high on your toes, keeping your back straight, chest high, and eyes looking forward.
- Pause for a second.

E-Centric Phase

- 1-2-3-4-5-6-down. Slowly, lower yourself back down to the step, allowing your heel to drop below the step for an extra stretch.
- Repeat the exercise.
- Reverse the position and repeat with your right leg.

Pointers

- Don't let your hips move backward or forward.
- Don't bend at the knee; this creates momentum and takes away from the effectiveness of the exercise.
- Rise up as high as possible on each repetition and flex your calf muscles. You should be standing on your toes at the height of the exercise.

EXERCISE 7: SQUAT WITH DUMBBELLS

The squat strengthens the back, thighs, buttocks (glutei maximi), abdomen, and calf muscles. There are no more important ligaments to strengthen than those that support the knee, which is why it's critical that you have strong, powerful leg muscles. You'll appreciate it when you get out of a chair, go up stairs, walk, and run.

Get Set

- Hold a dumbbell in each hand at arm's length with the weights at your side, palms facing in.
- Keep your head up, knees slightly bent, back straight, and feet planted firmly on the floor, shoulder width apart.

E-Centric Phase

- 1-2-3-4-5-6-down. Slowly bend your knees until your upper thighs are almost parallel with the floor by the sixth second.
- As you descend, make sure that your buttocks move backward, which will keep your knees behind or just over your ankle joints, preventing knee strain.
- Hold the position for one second.

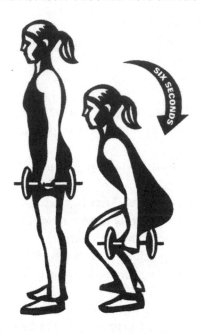

Upward Movement

- 1-2-up. Squeeze your buttocks as you return to the starting position.
- Repeat.

Pointers

- Be sure to keep your feet flat on the floor to prevent knee strain. If this is difficult—especially true for taller exercisers—use a wider stance.
- Your knees are under extreme pressure with this exercise, so do not let them move out beyond your toes or you will risk injury.
- Keep your back flat as you descend and ascend. Don't slump your shoulders or arch your back.
- When you push to come back up, push through with your heels rather than your toes.

EXERCISE 8:
FORWARD LUNGE WITH DUMBBELLS

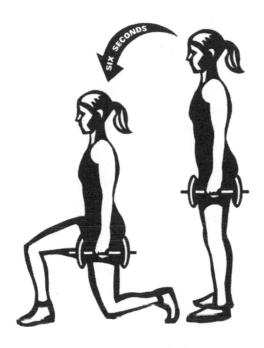

You know from Level One E-Centrics that the forward lunge firms and strengthens your buttocks, the quadriceps on the front of your thighs, the hamstrings on the back of your thighs, and your calves.

Get Set

- Standing, hold a dumbbell in each hand, with your arms hanging by your sides and the weights at your side, palms facing in.
- Keep your head up, back straight, and feet planted firmly on the floor, about fourteen inches apart.
- Slowly take an exaggerated step forward with your right foot as far as possible, keeping your back straight, chest high, chin up, eyes looking forward.

E-Centric Phase

- 1-2-3-4-5-6-down. Slowly bend your right knee to a 90-degree angle (your thigh is almost parallel with the floor) so your right knee is now over your right ankle.

- Lower your left knee until it is a few inches from the ground. Your left heel will rise off the floor. Do not let your left knee rest on the floor.
- Balance your weight on your right heel and the toes of your left foot.
- Pause for a second.

Upward Movement

- 1-2-up. Slowly step back to the start position by straightening your right leg, pushing off from your heel.
- Step forward with your left foot.
- Repeat.

Pointers

- To maintain proper balance, step straight forward, with your feet shoulder width apart.
- Lunge only as far forward as you can while still maintaining your balance.
- Don't look down.
- Don't shift your weight forward. Be sure to keep it directly over your hips to prevent excess pressure on your knees.
- Don't let your knees roll inward or let them bow outward. This will overstress your knees.
- Don't round your back. This may overstress your lower back.

Level Two Overview

This month's goal is to complete three E-Centric workouts per week. No excuses! The exercises are modified from those you learned last month, so there will be no surprises. What I want you to do is to aim for weight increases of at least 5 percent in each of the eight exercises by the end of the month. It's going to take some perseverance and concentration on your part. Give it your best shot. You've got nothing to lose but body fat and lots to gain, such as increased muscle and a healthy boost of self-confidence. Go for it!

As you would expect, the weight-training sessions become more challenging when you move from your own body weight for resistance and add the dumbbells. But the major metabolic boost is well worth the effort.

At the end of Week 8, take your measurements again, and have your photos taken. I'm sure you've seen some improvement. I'm sure you're standing taller now and move with more grace and power. And you probably have some added spring in your step.

If you're not on target, don't worry. Stick with the AstroFit plan, and your body will respond sooner rather than later. That's my guarantee. Renew your vow to yourself that you are going to achieve your goals. You are going to use your dumbbells three times a week. You are going to perform your aerobic exercise at least three times a week. It will all be worth it. Before you know, you will be achieving your goals. You'll become stronger and fitter. Your clothes will fit better. And you will have reversed the aging process, making you younger than you were when you started your AstroFit program three months ago!

9

Level Three E-Centrics: At the Gym

What saves a man is to take a step. Then another step.
—ANTOINE DE SAINT-EXUPÉRY

When I think about gyms and health clubs, I recall the dozens of airy, spacious clubs I've had the pleasure of exercising in over the years. With row upon row of gleaming chrome and steel weight machines awaiting my use—each specifically designed to strengthen a particular body part—these gyms offered an efficient and safe way to build muscle.

I like to work out on machines, and I appreciate their advantages. With my time often at a premium, I get my exercise done with no time spent bending to slip weighted iron plates onto the Olympic bar or looking for matched dumbbells. Instead, all I do is pull out a steel pin on a weight stack machine, slip it into the slot of the number of pounds that I want to lift, align myself on the bench, and start exercising.

With Keiser strength equipment, it's even easier. Simply press a button, and the resistance is incrementally increased or decreased with compressed air. Moving from machine to machine, after thirty or so sweat-drenched minutes I've given myself a total-body workout. I've stressed myself for the day, but it's a good stress and I feel great. In the process, I've added more life to my years—and years to my life—and as I head back to work or home, I have a nice bounce to my step.

Weight Machines

Following are some of the advantages of working with weight machines:

- *Safety.* Machines offer the safest way to exercise with weights. On quality machines, the heavy weight stacks are held by pulleys and cables and locked into a track. If you can no longer lift the load or for some reason you have to let go, you can do so without fear of having the weights come crashing down.
- *Muscle isolation.* Some machines are better than free weights at isolating specific muscle groups that you may want to exercise.
- *Efficiency.* Weight machines offer efficiency of time and space. Since you can perform as many as seventy different weight routines on some quality multistation machines just by moving a cable or pulling a pin, your time is spent exercising rather than taking weight plates off the bar and putting them back on.
- *Proper form.* Machines enforce proper lifting patterns. As you push or pull the weights, the machine guides you along a predetermined, fixed track, making it impossible to develop an incorrect lifting form.

There are a few disadvantages as well:

- *Lack of specificity.* The machines lock you into a particular movement pattern. This is a disadvantage for more serious exercisers because the machine develops only the large muscle groups, ignoring the smaller supporter muscles that aid in developing overall power and strength.
- *One size does not fit all.* Not all machines fit all body sizes. If you are over six feet or under five feet tall, you may feel cramped or stretched on some machines. This prevents you from being able to assume the proper body position for each exercise and limits your ability to move the machine's levers or grips far enough to perform the exercise properly.

Choosing a Gym

With so many gyms now open in most cities, where to exercise is no longer a problem. If you want to go the health club route, your timing could not be better. Club membership is soaring nationally, especially in the over-thirty age category. The more select clubs focus on service, programs, and qualified staff and you pay for them, but this often leads to exercise adherence. Less expensive, high-volume clubs will make up for lack of amenities and classes with plenty of sophisticated high-tech equipment.

Write down your specific needs and check them off as you inspect the facility. Before signing on for anything, be sure to take the following ten steps:

Step 1: Shop around. Come up with a list of clubs within fifteen minutes of home or work. Any farther away, and the odds of your using the facility regularly are slim. Ask friends if they know anything about the clubs you're considering. Don't forget about the Y and community centers.

Step 2: Ask for a complimentary twenty-four-hour workout pass. This way you can experience the club for a day. If the salesperson doesn't offer this, purchase a day pass; it's money well spent. When deciding on whether or not you want to go the club route, I strongly recommend that you take advantage of the free one- to two-week trial memberships that most clubs now offer.

Step 3: Make sure the club has a welcoming attitude to people of all ages and fitness levels. Many beginning exercisers feel like the proverbial fish out of water when walking into a health club. It's up to the staff to make sure that you feel at home. Are the instructors helpful in getting you started on your program? Do they seem friendly and readily offer helpful training advice and encouragement?

Step 4: Visit the club at a time when you think you'd work out. Whether it's 7 A.M. or 7 P.M., you want to know who you will be sharing the space with. You will also get a clear idea of how crowded it will be when you plan to exercise. The last thing you want to do is have to stand in line waiting to get onto a particular machine.

Step 5: Make sure the club provides a safe environment. Are staff
members certified in CPR (cardiopulmonary resuscitation) and
ready to administer other forms of emergency aid? Are the fitness
instructors certified by a nationally recognized organization?
These groups include the American College of Sports Medicine
(ACSM), the National Fitness Academy (NFA), and the
International Dance Exercise Association (IDEA).

Step 6: Make sure there is enough equipment available. The facility
should have the type and quantity of equipment that will enable
you to meet your goals. If you want weight-stack machines but
the gym mainly has free weights, then it's not for you. And
having to wait for a machine becomes a great excuse to skip the
workout and head for the shower.

*Step 7: Don't forget about your aerobic workouts. Find out how many
pieces of aerobic equipment are available.* This includes stair
climbers, treadmills, elliptical trainers, rowing machines, and
stationary bikes. Are there sufficient cardiofitness classes that
interest you that meet at convenient times? Is there a lap pool,
or does the club have water aerobics classes?

Step 8: Ask about child care possibilities. It's better to bring your
child to the gym with you than miss your workout. Many clubs
offer baby-sitting service. Be sure to check hours and price.

Step 9: Note the details. They may be small, but they're important.
Is there music playing that will enhance your workouts? Or is it
loud and intrusive and will drive you to distraction? Does the
gym sparkle? Is the locker room clean? Does the club really offer
the ambience that's going to let you get the best workouts
possible?

Step 10: Be ready to discuss price. Leave your credit card and
checkbook at home so there will be no pressure to sign on during
the first visit. The salesperson may tell you that the "special"
sales price ends that afternoon, but don't be bullied. Be wary
about signing any kind of contract until you know what it
stipulates. Read every word and ask exactly what it is that the
contract requires and exactly how much you will have to pay.
Don't be afraid to ask questions. Some clubs have monthly fees;
others require an initiation fee, plus monthly dues. Some

contracts lock you in for as long as two or more years, with a penalty if you leave early. Note whether or not there are any extra fees for other services. For example, is there an extra charge for the sauna, hot tub, pool, and laundry service?

Working with a Personal Trainer

You've undoubtedly read about the personal trainers to the stars making headlines for helping Hollywood's "A list" look healthy and taut, preventing pro athletes from getting fat, and helping high-profile corporate execs achieve the body shape and fitness level they need to keep their image-conscious jobs. But in reality, most personal trainers work with ordinary people who lack the motivation or know-how they need to exercise regularly and efficiently on their own.

Although using a trainer may seem a luxury—trainer fees range from $20 an hour to ten times that amount in some parts of the country—handing over your money to someone to instruct, prod, and inspire you may prove to be one of your better investments.

Clients generally exercise in the privacy of their own home and use their own equipment, if they have any, or else work against the resistance supplied by the trainer. In some instances, a client works out with the trainer in a local health club. Be sure of your obligations beforehand so you won't be surprised by any extra fees for your session.

Paying a personal trainer to make you sweat is ultimately your choice—and your money. In the end, you may not come out looking like a Hollywood star, but if you end up working out regularly with a trainer and feel like a star because of it, who could ask for anything more?

E-Centric Exercises with Weight Machines

The gym version of the AstroFit program consists of eight exercises—seven on various machines, plus the Cobra. Together, they will give you a complete body workout.

The instructions I've provided are general but will apply to most pieces of equipment you'll see. Before starting, make sure that you understand how to use the equipment properly. If the gym you use doesn't have the equipment I've described here, ask the trainer to suggest a suitable replacement exercise.

The following training tips will help you achieve maximum gains from your E-Centric workouts at the gym.

Don't try to be Superman or Wonder Woman. Do not overload your
weight machine. If this is your first time with machine weights,
or if you haven't been to the gym in a while, experiment with
different weights to see how they feel. Know your physical
limitations. Overexertion can lead to injury and setbacks in your
training. *Choose a weight that seems comfortable for the movement
you want to do; then use half of it.* In your early workouts you
should be working with light weight at 10 to 15 repetitions. This
way you'll condition your joints without damaging them and
you'll be able to learn proper lifting technique.

Proper warm-ups are critical. Running, riding your exercise bike,
skipping rope, or using a stair climber, ski machine, or rower are
some of the ways to get your heart rate up and prepare your
muscles for the impending weight work. Don't forget to cool
down, too.

Breathe correctly when you lift. The correct way to breathe is to inhale
just before you lift and exhale slowly as you let the weights back
down. Never hold your breath when you lift weights because this
reduces the flow of blood back to your heart and subsequently
affects the blood flow to your brain. This may lead to light-
headedness and fainting, which could be especially dangerous if
you are performing an overhead exercise.

Take a moment to examine the equipment closely. Look over the cables,
pulleys, welded joints, and pads to make sure that they all appear
to be in perfect working order. Don't use a machine if any joint is
cracked or loose.

Be careful when changing weights. When changing weight loads, be
sure to place the selector key *completely* into the slot. Don't place

your fingers under the weight stack when removing the key. Also, keep your fingers away from any pulleys, levers, cams, or belts.

Level Three E-Centric Exercises with Weight Machines

1. Biceps curl with weight machine
2. Chest press with weight machine
3. "Lat" pull-down with weight machine
4. Abdominal crunch with weight machine
5. Cobra
6. Calf raise with weight machine
7. Leg press with weight machine
8. Hamstring curl with weight machine

EXERCISE 1:
BICEPS CURL WITH WEIGHT MACHINE
The biceps curl, like the at-home version with dumbbells, strengthens the muscles in the front of your upper arms and wrists.

Get Set
- Set the resistance.
- Adjust the seat height so that your back is erect, your feet are flat on the floor, and your triceps (the backs of your upper arms) rest comfortably on the pad.
- Extend your arms forward and grab the handles with your palms facing up.

Upward Movement
- 1-2-up. Slowly pull the grips and contract your biceps muscles until you raise your hands to the level of your face. Your triceps must remain on the pads.
- Pause for a second.

E-Centric Phase
- 1-2-3-4-5-6-down. Slowly lower your arms to the starting position.
- Repeat the exercise.

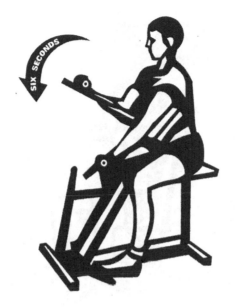

Pointers

- Make sure the seat is properly adjusted. If it is too high or too low, you will strain your shoulders or elbows.
- To maintain emphasis on the biceps, be sure to keep your triceps on the pads as you lift and lower.
- Maintain an erect posture. Do not tilt your head and shoulders down to help raise or lower the weights; this makes the curl less effective. If you can't lift the weight for each repetition without doing some kind of gyration, reduce the weight and repeat.

EXERCISE 2:
CHEST PRESS WITH WEIGHT MACHINE

This exercise works your chest muscles, as well as your shoulders and triceps.

Get Set

- Set the resistance.
- Adjust the seat so the center of your chest lines up with the handles.
- Grip the handles with your palms facing out, elbows at your sides.

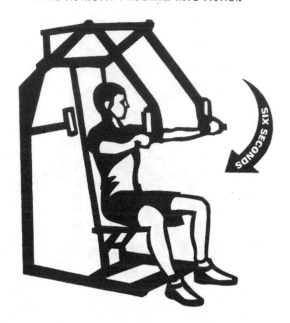

Upward Movement

- 1-2-up. Push the handles forward until your arms are straight.
- Pause for a second.
  ### E-Centric Phase
- 1-2-3-4-5-6-down. Slowly lower the handles back to the starting position.
- Repeat.
  ### Pointer
- Keep good form with your neck and back firmly against the back-rest.

EXERCISE 3:
"LAT" PULL-DOWN WITH WEIGHT MACHINE

The "lat" pull-down strengthens the biceps of the upper arm and the big latissimus dorsi muscles of your back that sweep along both sides of your rib cage. In this exercise, the E-Centric movement comes from resisting the pull of the weights *upward*.

Get Set

- Set the resistance.
- Sit down so you are facing the machine, feet flat on the floor.

- Adjust the seat so your knees are at a 90-degree angle to the floor.
- Grab the overhead bar with an overhand grip, hands slightly wider than shoulder width apart, palms facing forward.

Downward Movement

- 1-2-down. Slowly pull the bar down.
- Lean back slightly, squeezing your shoulder blades together as the bar comes toward your chest.
- Pause for a second.

E-Centric Phase

- 1-2-3-4-5-6-up. Slowly resist as the bar raises back up to the top position.
- Repeat.

Pointers

- Don't pull the bar behind your back. This could damage the rotator cuff muscles of your shoulder.
- Keep your back straight; if you have to bend forward in order to lower the weight, you're using too heavy a weight. Reduce the load and repeat.

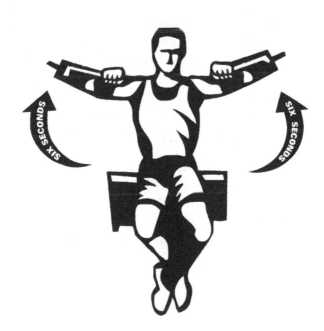

EXERCISE 4:
ABDOMINAL CRUNCH WITH WEIGHT MACHINE

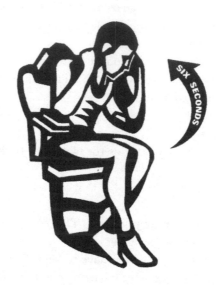

When performed properly, this exercise effectively isolates the front abdominal muscle (rectus abdominis). Leaning forward and pushing against the resistance of the machine compresses your abdominal muscles. The powerful E-Centric portion of this exercise comes from resisting the weights as they go back to the starting position.

Get Set

- Set the resistance.
- Adjust the seat so your upper thighs are parallel to the floor.
- Grab the overhead handles and position your triceps on the pads.

Downward Movement

- 1-2-down. Contract your abdominal muscles and lean forward so your shoulders come closer to your hips.
- Pause for a second.

E-Centric Phase

- 1-2-3-4-5-6-up. Resist the upward pull as you slowly return to the starting upright position.

Pointer

- Don't put on so much weight that you can barely bend over. Adjust accordingly.

EXERCISE 5: COBRA

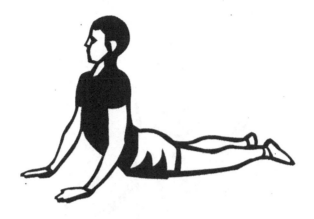

As you already know from your Level One and Level Two work-outs, this classic yoga exercise helps to gently stretch and strengthen the muscles of your lower back and hips, as well as your upper arms.

Get Set

- Lie on your stomach with your face almost touching the mat.
- Place your palms on the mat at the sides of your shoulders.
- Keep your legs together and the tops of your feet resting on the mat.

Upward Movement

- 1-2-3-4-up. Push up, bringing your head up off the mat.
- Keep your pelvis pushed into the mat while relaxing your buttocks as best you can.
- Slowly arch your spine backward, straightening your elbows.
- Bring your head back and look at the ceiling.
- Pause for a second.

E-Centric Phase

- 1-2-3-4-5-6-down. Descend slowly to the mat, then repeat.

Pointers

- Keep your back relaxed.
- Let your arms do the work as you rise up and descend back to the mat. Don't hunch your shoulders together.
- If you're unable to lift up and straighten your arms, begin the exercise propped up on your elbows.

EXERCISE 6:
CALF RAISE WITH WEIGHT MACHINE

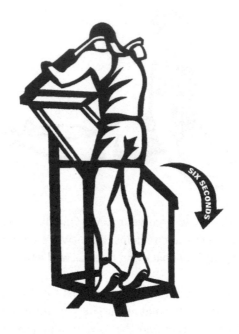

This exercise targets your gastrocnemius muscles (calves), and when performed through a full range of motion, it is one of the most effective exercises for enhancing the strength of these important muscles.

Get Set

- Set the resistance.
- Place the balls of your feet on the edge of the platform shoulder width apart so that your heels are projecting over the edge.
- Position your shoulders under the padded movement levers.
- Straighten your legs so you are standing upright.

Upward Movement

- 1-2-up. Rise up on your toes as high as you can, flexing your calves.
- Pause for a second.

E-Centric Phase

- 1-2-3-4-5-6-down. Slowly descend to the platform until your heels are below parallel on the platform.
- Repeat.

Pointers
- The key to great form in this exercise is getting the full range of motion, going as high and as low as you can.
- Keep your legs straight the entire time.

EXERCISE 7:
LEG PRESS WITH WEIGHT MACHINE

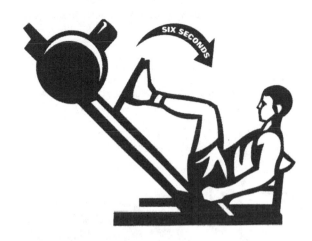

The leg press strengthens the muscles of your upper legs: buttocks, quadriceps, and hamstrings.

Get Set
- Set the resistance.
- Adjust the foot plate so that when you sit your back is snug against the back rest.
- Your knees should be bent so they are almost 90 degrees to the foot plate.
- Place your feet on the foot plate hip width apart, toes pointing upward, heels directly behind the toes.
- Grab the handles.

Outward Movement
- 1-2-up. Slowly push against the platform with your *heels* until your legs are almost straight.
- Pause for a second.

E-Centric Phase

- 1-2-3-4-5-6-down. Slowly lower the weights by bending your knees and moving back to the starting position.
- Repeat.

Pointers

- Don't bend your legs so far that your thighs end up pushing against your chest. This puts undue pressure on your knee joints.
- When extending your legs in the outward portion of the exercise, don't fully straighten your legs and lock your knees. This puts too much pressure on the knee joints.

EXERCISE 8:
HAMSTRING CURL WITH WEIGHT MACHINE

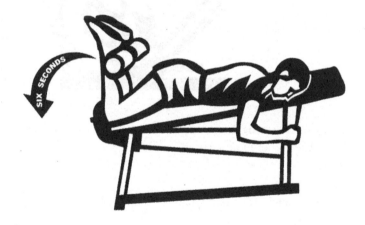

This exercise is one of the most effective ways of strengthening your hamstring muscles. If they are neglected in training, it leads to an imbalance between the front and back of the thigh. To protect against knee injury, it's important to develop both sides.

Get Set

- Select the resistance.
- Lie on your stomach on the bench.

- Position your knees so they are just off the edge of the bench. You know that you are positioned correctly if the ankle pad now rests comfortably on your ankle—not your calf or heel.
- Hold the handles.

Upward Movement

- 1-2-up. Bend your knees until they are fully bent and your heels are as close to your buttocks as possible.
- Pause for a second.

E-Centric Phase

- 1-2-3-4-5-6-down. Slowly lower your legs, straightening them out until they are fully extended.
- Repeat.

Pointers

- To avoid knee pain, make sure that your knees are over the edge of the bench.
- Keep your hips pressed into the bench. Don't arch your back to help curl the weight up. This will not isolate the hamstrings and may end up hurting your lower back.

10

E-Centrics with a Partner

A man's health can be judged by which he takes two at a time: pills or the stairs.
—JOAN WELSH

In this world where everything, including exercise equipment, seems to have a computer chip embedded within it, it's amazing the kind of beneficial E-Centric workout you can get from just pulling against a towel or by having a friend gently push against your shoulders to supply resistance. Exercising with a training partner is a way to make substantial and impressive gains in lean muscle mass. For these eight basic exercises, no equipment is necessary. Just grab a sturdy towel from your linen closet, and you're all ready to go.

Exercising with a motivated partner can enhance your workouts immensely. Because few people train as intensely as they think they do, your partner can gauge how much effort you're putting into the workout and give you a lot of positive encouragement to help boost your exercise intensity. By providing the necessary resistance as he or she pulls against the towel you're holding, your partner can also help you to work just a little harder.

The beauty of these E-Centric workouts is that all your partner—whether your friend, wife, husband, significant other, or child—has to do is supply resistance. The fun quotient will begin to rise as soon as you both get the hang of what's expected in each exercise.

It's up to your partner to allow the movements of the particular exercise to occur in a smooth fashion, while supplying just enough resistance so that the movement is sufficiently difficult to perform. Your partner's goal is to make sure the resistance is steady right through to the final sixth second of each E-Centric phase.

Perform one set of ten repetitions for each exercise. If your partner is also going to be working out, switch off after each set so you alternate providing the resistance.

E-Centric Exercises with a Partner

1. Biceps curl with partner
2. Lateral arm descent with partner
3. Triceps extension with partner
4. Overhead shoulder press with partner
5. Push-up with partner—modified and classic
6. Sit-up with partner
7. Knee curl with partner

EXERCISE 1: BICEPS CURL WITH PARTNER

The biceps curl strengthens the muscles in the front of your upper arm and wrists.

Get Set
- Kneel on the floor.
- Keep your elbows close to your body and flex your elbows until your forearms and hands are parallel to the floor.
- Have your partner stand in front of you and place his palms on yours.

Upward Movement
- 1-2-up. As your partner resists, slowly raise your palms upward toward your chest.

E-Centric Phase
- 1-2-3-4-5-6-down. Have your partner press down on your palms as you resist the downward push until your forearms are parallel to the floor.
- Pause and repeat.

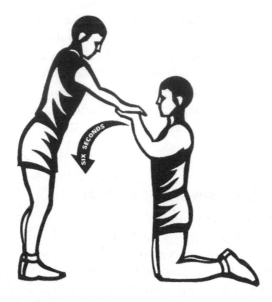

Pointers

- To maintain emphasis on the biceps, be sure to keep your elbows firmly in place against your sides as you lower and lift.
- Do not swing your body to help raise your arms.
- Always look straight ahead as you curl. When you look down, your shoulders automatically hunch forward, making the curl less effective.

EXERCISE 2:
LATERAL ARM DESCENT WITH PARTNER

The lateral arm descent strengthens your shoulder muscles.

Get Set

- Stand with your arms at your sides, feet shoulder width apart.
- Raise your arms laterally to shoulder height, palms facing down so they are parallel to the floor.
- Have your partner stand behind you with his or her hands on your forearms.

E-Centric Phase

- 1-2-3-4-5-6-down. Slowly begin to lower your arms as your partner presses down on your forearms.
- Resist this motion as you lower your arms to your sides.

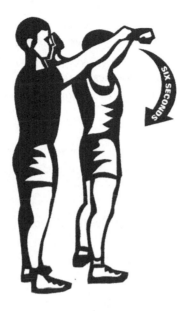

Upward Movement

• 1-2-up. As your partner resists, raise your arms to the starting position and repeat.

Pointers

• Keep your back straight.
• Do not bend your head; look forward the entire time.

EXERCISE 3:
TRICEPS EXTENSION WITH PARTNER

The triceps extension strengthens muscles in back of the upper arm and shoulders.

Get Set

• Stand with your back straight, your head up, and your feet on the floor, about sixteen inches apart.
• Hold the middle of a rolled-up towel in your hands.
• Raise your arms straight overhead.
• Have your partner stand behind you and hold on to the ends of the towel.
• Tense your abdominal muscles and look forward, keeping your head upright.

E-Centric Phase

- 1-2-3-4-5-6-down. As your partner pulls the towel down, resist and slowly lower your arms by bending them at the elbow but keeping your upper arms vertical throughout the exercise.
- Keep lowering the towel until your forearms and biceps touch.
- Pause for a second.

Upward Movement

- 1-2-up. As your partner supplies resistance, slowly raise the towel back to the starting position.
- Repeat.

Pointers

- When raising and lowering the towel, don't sway or arch your back.
- Don't allow your upper arms to move.

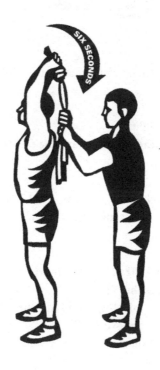

EXERCISE 4:
OVERHEAD SHOULDER PRESS WITH PARTNER

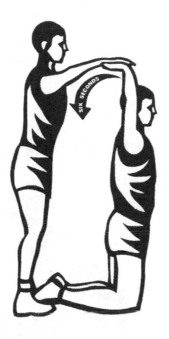

The overhead shoulder press strengthens the trapezius and del-toid muscles of the upper back as well as the triceps at the back of the upper arm.

Get Set
- Stand erect with your feet flat on the floor shoulder width apart.
- Keep your hands in front of your shoulders, palms facing up.
- Raise your arms so your hands are straight up over your head, palms facing up.
- Have your partner stand behind you and place his palms on yours.

E-Centric Phase
- 1-2-3-4-5-6-down. As your partner presses down on your palms, resist as you slowly lower your arms, bending your elbows so your hands finish up just behind your ears.
- Pause for a second.

Upward Movement
- 1-2-up. With your partner supplying resistance, slowly raise your arms straight back to the starting position.
Pointers
- Maintain perfect posture throughout the movements.
- Don't arch your back as you raise your arms upward. If you find yourself struggling to raise your arms, have your partner supply less resistance.

EXERCISE 5:
MODIFIED PUSH-UP WITH PARTNER

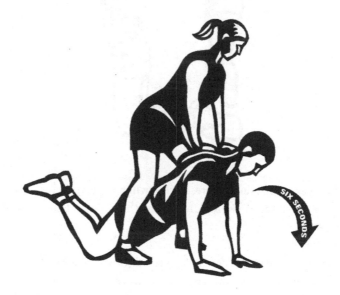

The push-up will strengthen your chest, shoulders, triceps, abdomen, and back muscles.
Get Set
- Get down on all fours on an exercise mat or rug with your arms extended, palms flat on the floor, shoulder width apart, fingers pointing forward. Your knees should be bent at slightly more than a 90-degree angle.

- Keep your feet perpendicular to the floor. They can also be extended in the air; do not cross them, or you will put extra pressure on your lower back.
- Have your partner straddle your lower back, standing with knees bent, feet flat on the floor, and hands on your shoulder blades.

E-Centric Phase

- 1-2-3-4-5-6-down. With your partner applying steady pressure on your shoulders, resist as you slowly lower yourself to the floor, touching the floor with your chin.
- Your chest, abdomen, and thighs should not touch the floor.
- Pause one second.

Upward Movement

- 1-2-up. With your partner applying steady pressure, straighten your arms out, keep your back flat, and, using your knees as the pivot point, push your upper legs and chest away from the floor and rise slowly back to the starting position.

Pointers

- Lower and lift your body as a single unit.
- Don't let your abdomen sag.

EXERCISE 5: CLASSIC PUSH-UP WITH PARTNER

If you've built enough strength and find the modified push-up to be too easy, perform this classic version instead.

Get Set

- Lie face down on the floor, your legs together.
- Keep your hands at the sides of your chest, palms flat on the floor.
- Raise your body onto your toes and hands, with your hands perpendicular to your shoulders.
- Have your partner stand with knees bent, feet flat on the floor, straddling your lower back, with her hands on your shoulder blades.

E-Centric Phase

- 1-2-3-4-5-6-down. With your partner applying steady pressure on your shoulders, resist as you slowly lower yourself to the floor, touching the floor with your chin.
- Your chest, abdomen, and thighs should not touch the floor.
- Pause one second.

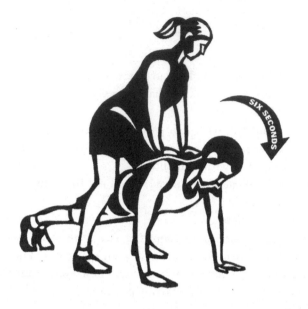

Upward Movement
- 1-2-up. With your partner applying steady pressure on your shoulders, exhale as you push back up to the starting position and repeat.

Pointer
- Don't continue if you feel any pain or strain in your lower back.

EXERCISE 6: SIT-UP WITH PARTNER
The sit-up strengthens the upper and lower abdominal muscles.

Get Set
- Lie on your back with your knees bent and your feet flat on the floor.
- Fold your arms across your chest.
- Have your partner kneel next to you and place his arms on your forearms.

Upward Movement
- 1-2-up. As you slowly lift your shoulders off the floor, have your partner supply light pressure.
- Stop when you reach 45 degrees and pause for a second.

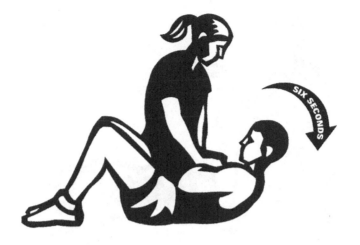

E-Centric Phase

- 1-2-3-4-5-6-down. Slowly return to the starting position, resisting the pressure exerted by your partner. Repeat.
Pointer
- Be sure to keep your feet flat on the floor.

EXERCISE 7: KNEE CURL WITH PARTNER
Get Set
- Lie on your stomach on the floor or an exercise mat or bench.
- Flex your knees so your heels touch your buttocks.
- Have your partner grab your lower leg just above your heels.
E-Centric Phase
- 1-2-3-4-5-6-down. Slowly lower your legs to the mat, with your partner supplying enough resistance that it takes six seconds to get to the mat.
- Pause for a second.
Upward Movement
- 1-2-up. With your partner supplying resistance, bend your knees until they are fully bent and your heels are as close to your buttocks as possible.
- Repeat.

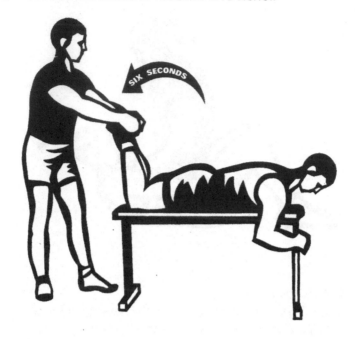

Pointers

- Keep your hips pressed into the mat.
- Don't arch your back to help curl your legs back up. You may hurt your lower back.

Four

Protecting Bone/Enhancing Balance

11

Building Healthy Bones

Prevention is better than cure.
—ERASMUS

Just as a muscle gets stronger and bigger the more you exercise, a bone becomes stronger and denser when stress is regularly placed on it. But when your bones are not called upon to help lift or perform other types of physical activity, they don't receive regular cellular messages telling them they need to be strong, and they soon begin to reduce their daily building processes. Over time, they become less dense and more prone to fracture.

Remember the twenty-eight-day bed-rest study I described in Chapter 2? The test subjects who do no exercise whatsoever during their four weeks in bed will lose *two years' worth* of calcium from their bones. This will confirm what we already knew from studies of Russian cosmonauts on various space missions: that inactivity is bad for bones.

In the 1970s, cosmonauts in microgravity used their arms extensively for working in the spaceship but used their legs very little. They lost bone mass from their lower vertebrae, hips, and thigh bones at a rate close to 1 percent per month for every month aloft. This rate of accelerated bone loss was ten times as high as that of osteoporosis, the abnormal thinning of the bones here on Earth that causes bones to become more fragile and more likely to break.

Bone loss has caused great concern in the space research community, especially in light of the fact that more than twenty years after their long missions, some of the Russian cosmonauts still have not regained their normal bone mass. Astronauts heading to Mars could potentially lose 30 to 60 percent of their calcium during the voyage, leaving their bones in a dangerously weakened state. In addition to developing weakened bones, they would be at high risk for developing painful kidney stones due to all the calcium being leached from their bones.

NASA has been addressing this problem. Nutrition, vitamins, and hormones will all play an important role in preventing serious bone depletion. A complete total-body E-Centric exercise program will be critical to maintaining each astronaut's bone mass.

The Body's Ongoing Bone-Making Process

Bone is a complex tissue that provides support for your muscles, protects your vital organs, and acts as the storehouse of calcium, the mineral essential for bone density. More than 90 percent of the body's supply of calcium is found in the bones.

Your skeleton has two distinct types of bones. *Cortical* bone, which is hard, dense, stiff, and designed to withstand stress, makes up about 80 percent of the skeleton. Cortical bone is found on the outer shell of most bones, in your hips, and in the long bones of your arms and legs. *Trabecular* bone, the second type of bone, is found within the cortical casings, in parts of your hips, at the ends of the long bones of your arms and legs, and in the vertebrae.

Throughout life, living bone undergoes a continuous process of breaking down and building up, a complex procedure known as *re-modeling*. Bones remodel themselves in order to grow and to repair any minor damage that may have occurred during the day. When bones are remodeling, old bone is removed and replaced by new bone.

Remodeling starts when a variety of chemicals in the body direct bone-eroding cells, known as *osteoclasts,* to break down and remove bone in a process known as *bone resorption.* This releases small amounts of calcium, magnesium, and phosphorous into the bloodstream. At the same time, other chemicals—the hormone estrogen, especially—send messages to bone cells known as *osteoblasts*, directing them to make new bone. First they fill in with collagen the tiny cavities made by the osteoclasts, and then they lay down new calcium, magnesium, and phosphorus extracted from the bloodstream until the bone surface is completely restored.

Osteoporosis: The Silent Thief

It's estimated that as much as 10 to 30 percent of the adult skeleton is remodeled each year, keeping the bones strong and dense. Bones achieve their maximum strength and density around the age of twenty. This level remains stable for a few years and then slowly begins to decrease. On average, an adult loses about 1 percent of total bone mass every year.

When women reach menopause, the osteoclast/osteoblast balance gets out of sync due to the loss of estrogen and progesterone. Bone loss increases significantly to upward of 3 percent annually during this period. If this loss continues unabated, it may result in osteoporosis.

Meaning "porous bones" in Latin, osteoporosis is the silent thief that robs people of their bone strength without showing any initial symptoms. After someone falls or has an accident, the bone loss quickly becomes apparent. Even a minor fall can break a weakened wrist, forearm, or vertebrae of the spine.

Although osteoporosis can affect both men and women, it's about eight times as common in women. According to the National Osteoporosis Foundation, a woman's risk of developing an osteoporosis-related injury is equal to her *combined* risk of developing breast, ovarian, or uterine cancer.

Many women think they don't have to start worrying about osteoporosis until menopause, but this is a mistake. It's also a mistake for men to believe they don't have to worry about this bone disease. It appears that osteoporosis is more prevalent in men than had been thought, and the main cause is now thought to be the same for both sexes: an age-related drop in estrogen, the female sex hormone that's also found in low levels in men. It's now estimated that of the

10 million Americans who have osteoporosis, more than 1.5 million are men, and that one in eight men age fifty and older develop osteoporosis-related fractures.

Diagnosing Osteoporosis

Just as a blood pressure test can assess your risk of hypertension, a painless and noninvasive bone density test can indicate your risk of bone fracture. Since peak bone density is reached between the ages of thirty and forty and then begins to fall, women should have their first bone density test when their menstrual periods become irregular or other perimenopausal symptoms begin.

Dual-energy X-ray absorptiometry, or DEXA, is the most common bone density test used today. This involves lying on a padded table for ten minutes while a special X-ray machine scans your spine, hips, or forearm using ultralow X-ray levels to precisely determine bone mass. This invaluable screening tool, which can detect even a 1 percent change in bone density, is the "gold standard" of bone density measurement.

Peripheral dual-energy X-ray absorptiometry, or pDEXA, is a portable version of the DEXA machine that is now regularly used to measure bone density in the heel, finger, or wrist.

With both devices, a score is determined that tells how strong your bones are in comparison to what is considered to be normal peak bone mass.

Protecting Your Bones

Many factors influence bone growth. Your daily intake of calcium, vitamin D, protein, and other nutrients affects the health of your bones. The sex hormones—testosterone *and* estrogen in men, and estrogen in women—are a major influence on calcium uptake by bone tissue, and thus affect skeletal strength. Physical activity also plays a major role in bone growth and maintenance. When muscles work

Risk Factors for Osteoporosis

Some people are more liable to develop osteoporosis than others. The factors that increase your likelihood of developing the disease include:

- Being female; by age 65, the average woman retains slightly more than 74 percent of her bone mass, while most men have more than 90 percent
- Having osteoporosis in the family
- Being chronically underweight or having a slight, "small-boned" frame
- Early or surgical menopause before age 45
- In men, low testosterone levels (hypogonadism)
- A diet low in vitamins, calcium, and other minerals
- Being Caucasian or of Eurasian ancestry
- Smoking; this blocks the activity of estrogen and interferes with the maintenance of bone density
- Drinking more than three cups a day of coffee, cola, or tea
- Prolonged use of cortisone or prednisone
- Being sedentary and not performing strength-training and other forms of weight-bearing exercise

The more risk factors you have, the greater your chance of developing osteoporosis. If you have four or more of the common factors listed here, contact your physician and discuss having a bone density test to see whether you have osteoporosis or are likely to develop it in the future.

against gravity, the bones respond to the stress by becoming denser and stronger. This stress comes primarily from weight-bearing activity, such as walking and jogging, in which your legs support your body.

Over the years, I have designed research projects to examine strategies to keep us young and healthy. Following is some of the scientific evidence about bone health.

Protein and Bone Health

One of my earlier studies examined the effects of nutrition on bone health. The impetus for the study came from the fact that many young female athletes lose their menstrual cycles. Once menstruation stops, the release of the hormone estrogen is curtailed and bone remodeling ceases, leading to *osteopenia,* or low bone density. This explains why the bone density of female distance runners is often lower than that of women who perform no exercise at all.

In the past, many scientists speculated that the cessation of menstruation (a disorder called *amenorrhea*) was caused by abnormally low body fat levels. The thinking was that when a woman drops below a certain body fat level—12 percent or lower—the body perceives that pregnancy would be difficult, and amenorrhea sets in to prevent possible conception. Our study demonstrated that this was not true. Women with a low level of body fat are not doomed to amenorrhea.

A group of young female runners who ran at least twenty miles a week, and who had not menstruated for at least a year, were recruited and age-matched with a group of women who had perfectly normal menstrual cycles. To our surprise, we found that there was no difference in body fat percentages between the women. The runners and the control group both averaged about 20 percent body fat.

Upon close examination of their diets, however, it was determined that the active women were consuming 20 percent less protein and almost 500 fewer calories a day than their counterparts. My belief is that protein plays a huge part in bone health. Low protein intake, in addition to reducing the amount of body muscle, inhibits estrogen production, and estrogen is essential to bone production. With estrogen levels dropping, bone remodeling slows down significantly, and the body begins to undergo some sort of premature menopause.

When I examined the diet and body composition of a top female bodybuilder, she had a body fat percentage of 12. I discovered that even though this internationally ranked athlete was on a calorie-restricted diet, her bone density was absolutely normal and she was menstruating. Her weight training, combined with a high intake of protein, ensured the health of her bones as well as her overall good health.

Weight-Bearing Exercise and Bone Density

In order to determine if weight-bearing exercise (walking) conserves bone density in postmenopausal women, I recruited a group of women to participate in a one-year walking program. Half of the women walked at a brisk pace four days a week for fifty minutes, while the other half remained sedentary. After a year, the sedentary women had lost bone in their spine, while those women who walked regularly had not.

I think the bone-protecting effects of walking may have to do with its positive effect on trabecular bone, which is spongy and remodels more rapidly than cortical bone. Although the walking program did not *increase* bone density, these women were able to maintain their healthy bones. Given the number of crush fractures in the spine that are suffered each year, the fact that walking either slows or arrests fractures in the spine is a great bonus for regular walkers.

Walking is a fine activity, and if you have the time, it offers many other healthful benefits. For example, one eight-year study of nearly 73,000 women ages forty to sixty-five found that women who walked briskly for at least three hours each week had a 30 to 40 percent lower risk for heart attack than did sedentary women. The same risk reduction was found in women who exercised vigorously for ninety minutes per week, whether they were swimming laps, running, or doing aerobics.

When it comes to increasing bone density, however, walking and cardiovascular exercise pale in comparison to the multiple benefits accrued from weight training.

Strength Training and Bone Density

Based on all the positive effects of strength training that were emerging from my laboratory, I wondered if regular strength training would increase bone density. In fact, I had already noticed a striking relationship between muscle strength and bone density: women who were very weak also had the lowest bone density.

After receiving funding from the National Institutes of Health, I began a one-year strength-training study to examine the specific effects of strength training on bone density in postmenopausal women. Almost forty women between the ages of fifty and seventy were recruited for the trial. None was taking hormones. Half were to perform five high-intensity weight-training exercises twice a week, while the other group of women remained sedentary.

Many of the women who expressed some interest in an exercise program were initially skeptical about "weight lifting" and didn't want to commit themselves to something they perceived as masculine, vain, or both. What ultimately changed their minds was coming to my laboratory and seeing all of the women working out on our Keiser strength-training equipment. Their initial skepticism quickly vanished when they talked to the exercising women, who reported that not only was the exercise fun and made them feel great, but it had given them a complete body makeover they had never experienced before from any other type of exercise.

The final results of this study, which were published in *The Journal of the American Medical Association* in 1994, showed definitively that strength training has an effect on bone density. The exercising women gained an average of 1 percent in bone density. The sedentary women lost a pound of muscle and put on weight. They also lost 2.5 percent of their bone mass at the hip and spine, which is not uncommon in women during the first years after menopause.

In addition to increasing the density of their bones, the "weight-lifting" women gained three pounds of metabolically active muscle and lost three pounds of body fat. Most of them saw 75 percent increases in their overall strength. Although the women in this study strength-trained only twice a week, they were much more physically active at the end of the study than the sedentary women. In addition, gains of 14 percent in overall balance were noted in the strength-training group. Improved balance made these women less prone to falling and sustaining a fracture.

In addition to these benefits, strength training also increases production of peptides called IGF-1 (insulinlike growth factor–1). IGF-1 is used by the body for growth, metabolism, and survival. Furthermore, IGF-1 levels have a direct effect on bone remodeling.

AstroFit Bone-Building Strategies

Building strong bones early is like putting money in the bank. Inevitably you will need to withdraw, but how much is there to begin with determines how much will be left years later.

While as much as 30 percent of the skeleton is formed between the ages of nine and fourteen, science has proven that the restorative powers of strength training are remarkable at any age. Prevention of bone loss is much easier than treatment, and no matter what your age, you can still take steps to prevent bone loss.

Between Twenty and Thirty-five

Your bones will have reached their peak strength during these early adult years, so make sure you get plenty of calcium and perform your weekly E-Centric workouts.

Between Thirty-five and Fifty

Bone begins to gradually slow its overall remodeling process. To keep bone loss to a minimum during this time, perform E-Centrics and other weight-loading activities. Be sure to consume calcium-rich foods daily.

Women: If your menstrual periods become irregular or you develop signs of menopause such as hot flashes, consult with your doctor about hormone replacement treatment.

50 and Older

Perform your E-Centrics two to three times a week, and walk or jog for a half hour three times a week.

Women: If you have gone through menopause, you can lose as much as 6 percent of your bone mass per year. Speak to your doctor and see if hormone replacement with estrogen alone is an appropriate bone-protecting strategy for you, or if you are a candidate for a prescription medication for osteoporosis treatment.

The AstroFit Bone Protection Program

Even if you've waited until your forties, fifties, or sixties to start paying attention to the condition of your bones, there's still plenty of reason to follow this three-step preventive program. Your bones continue to evolve and change throughout your life. There's currently no cure for osteoporosis, but you can protect yourself with the following four-step AstroFit plan:

Step 1: Perform E-Centric and weight-bearing exercises
Step 2: Do the heel drop
Step 3: Get enough calcium
Step 4 (For women): Consider hormone replacement therapy

Step 1: Perform E-Centric and Weight-Bearing Exercises

E-Centric exercises are an excellent way to ensure optimal bone strength because they exert high forces on bone. Your bones respond to the added pressure by increasing in mass to spread the load over a larger amount of bone. Stress your bones regularly, and they will become denser and stronger. The beauty of the complete E-Centric program outlined in this book is that it builds muscle mass and strengthens bones all over the body.

A recent study conducted at the University of Oregon confirmed what I had believed for a long time about the bone-strengthening effects of weight training: if you don't use it, you lose it. In this study, researchers enrolled twenty-nine premenopausal women ages thirty-five to forty-five and had them perform strength-training exercises three times a week for a year. In addition to performing nine sets of ten squats and lunges (the same exercises you perform in the E-Centric training program), the women also did various jumping exercises, which put additional stress on their bones, especially the hips. As the study progressed, the women wore weighted vests to increase the stress on their bones even more.

When this phase of the study ended, bone density tests revealed that the women had made significant gains, increasing the bone mineral density of their thigh bones by as much as 3 percent. While this may not seem very much, consider that it translates to at least a 15 percent reduction in fracture risk.

In the second part of the study, the women "detrained" by not performing any resistance exercises for six months, then had their bone mineral density retested. The end result was that the women lost all the hard-earned gains accrued in their twelve months of strength training. By not having bone pulling on muscle three times a week, they lost the all-important cellular signal that was previously sent to remodel bone. To protect your bones, you will need to keep performing E-Centric exercises several times a week for the rest of your life.

Weight-bearing exercises are those in which your bones and muscles work against gravity, with your feet and legs bearing the weight. Walking, jogging, dancing, and aerobics are terrific weight-bearing activities for bone health. (They're also great for enhancing heart health and for helping with weight control.) On the other hand, swimming and bicycling are not the best weight-bearing activities for building bone density because the water and the bicycle tires—not your bones—are bearing most of your weight.

Step 2: Do the Heel Drop

When I met Professor Joan Bassey more than a decade ago at a conference in Baltimore, we began a lively discussion about our mutual research interests involving weight training and older people. I found Dr. Bassey, a physiologist from Nottingham, England, to be a solid investigator who was vitally interested in health and in discovering ways to slow down the aging processes with exercise.

With a little persuasion, she eventually agreed to spend a sabbatical year at my Center on Aging laboratory at Tufts University. Over the next twelve months, we carried out some interesting studies investigating how to enhance leg power and function in older people.

When Dr. Bassey returned home to Nottingham, she continued her own work, focusing most of her efforts on bone. Her aim was to find the simplest ways to enhance the overall strength of bone. Dr. Bassey has come up with a single exercise that protects against bone-thinning hot spots in the leg and hip. Her "heel drop" exercise—in which you rise up on your toes as high as possible and then let your heels drop forcefully back onto the floor—is so elementary and easy to perform that you can do heel drops anywhere, any time. Best of all, heel drops are guaranteed to make a significant difference in your bone density.

In her study, published in *Journal of Bone and Mineral Research*, Dr. Bassey examined the effects of heel drops on the bone density of the femur (thigh bone). At the beginning of the study, each participant had her bone density levels determined in order to establish a bone density baseline.

The first group of volunteers consisted of premenopausal women who performed a maximum of fifty heel drops, six days a week. When performed properly, each heel drop repetition was equal to the force of three times the person's body weight dropping onto the floor. The second group of volunteers consisted of postmenopausal women who performed the same exercise. A control group of women did no exercise at all.

Professor Bassey and her colleagues found that after five months, the heel drops resulted in a 3 percent jump in bone mineral density in the younger women. This significant bone boost, however, did not occur to the postmenopausal group performing the same exercise. Professor Bassey speculates that the reason for the differences between pre- and postmenopausal women may have to do with the quality of the bone.

Professor Bassey believes that heel drops are an easy way to preserve and increase bone mass in premenopausal women, and I wholeheartedly agree. If you are a premenopausal woman, I want you to perform this exercise five days a week. You don't have to perform all fifty repetitions at once but can break them up and do them throughout the day.

THE HEEL DROP

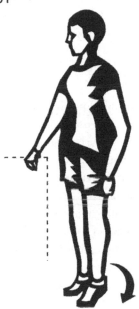

Perform fifty repetitions, either all at once or throughout the day. This exercise strengthens the bones of the leg, hip, thigh, and spinal column.

Get Set

- Remove your shoes.
- Stand at arm's length to the side of a wall with your back straight, and feet shoulder width apart.
- To ensure balance, touch the wall lightly with your fingertips.

Upward Movement

- Raise up high on your toes, keeping your back straight, chest high, and eyes looking forward.
- Pause for one second.

Downward Movement

- Keeping your hips and knees locked, let your heels drop to the floor, with your heels absorbing the full impact of the descent.
- Repeat the exercise.

Pointers

- Rise up as high as possible on each repetition.
- Don't let your hips move backward or forward.
- Don't bend at the knee; keep your legs straight.

Step 3: Get Enough Calcium

Calcium is the critical mineral needed to help build strong teeth and bones and to maintain bone density. Although most of the body's calcium is stored in the bones, the body doesn't produce its own supply; it comes from the food you consume. When there isn't enough calcium in your diet, your body extracts what it needs from your bones.

Evidence is unclear about the best dosage, but in general, the optimal amount of calcium depends on your age and personal risk factors. The daily recommended dietary allowance is 800 milligrams, except for adolescents and young adults (aged twelve to twenty-four) and pregnant or lactating women, who are advised to consume 1,200 milligrams daily. Some experts recommend that postmenopausal women consume at least 1,500 milligrams. Men should take 1,000 milligrams of calcium until age 65 and 1,500 milligrams in subsequent years.

Supplements of calcium may help maintain bone density and reduce the risk for a first fracture. One study reported that calcium plus vitamin D slowed bone loss in portions of the hips where a fracture is most serious.

CALCIUM-RICH FOODS

Many dark green leafy vegetables are rich sources of calcium, but the best source for most Americans, who usually don't eat enough veg-

The Calcium Content of Common foods

FOOD	PORTION	CALCIUM CONTENT (MG)
Salmon, with bones	1 can	484
Yogurt	1 cup, plain low-fat	415
Milk	1 cup, skim	315
Orange juice, calcium fortified	1 cup	300
Figs	10	270
Tofu, calcium fortified	4 ounces	260
Spinach	1 cup, cooked	245
Sesame seeds	1 cup	200
Kale	1 cup, cooked	95
Broccoli	1 cup, cooked	70
Almonds	1 ounce	80
Banana	1	10

etables, is low-fat or nonfat dairy products. The vitamin D added to milk and the lactose that occurs naturally in milk and dairy products are thought to aid in the absorption of calcium. It's best to get your calcium from food because it's most easily absorbed this way. If you can't get from your diet all the calcium you need, consider taking either a calcium carbonate or calcium nitrate supplement.

Step 4 (For Women): Consider Hormone Replacement Therapy

Natural hormone levels plummet at menopause. Hormone replacement therapy (HRT) consists of low-dose estrogen and progesterone. HRT can slow bone loss and prevent fractures, as well as reduce hot flashes and other common symptoms of menopause. The added progesterone in HRT also reduces the risk of endometrial cancer. HRT, if used to prevent osteoporosis, should be started at menopause for maximum effect.

While researchers are not sure of the long-term effects of HRT (over ten years), many believe that the benefits will be proved greater than the possible risks. Unfortunately, we won't have more definitive answers until at least 2007, the year when the Women's Health Ini-

Bone-Strengthening Nutrients

In addition to calcium, these are other important nutrients that are critical for bone health.

* *Vitamin C.* This powerful antioxidant, found in many fruits and vegetables, helps produce collagen, the important connective tissue that holds bone tissue together.
* *Vitamin D.* Without this vitamin, the bones cannot absorb or utilize calcium. Fortunately, we can make our own. Ten minutes of sunshine promote the manufacture of vitamin D in the body. Vitamin D–fortified milk is another good source.
* *Magnesium.* Found in green vegetables and nuts, this mineral is as important as calcium for overall bone strength and density.
* *Vitamin K.* Broccoli and leafy green vegetables, which are rich in this important vitamin, help promote the synthesis of three bone proteins essential for overall bone strength.
* *Potassium.* Found in fruits and vegetables, this mineral helps ensure that bones retain their calcium.

tiative study will be completed. This fifteen-year study—the largest study of women's health ever undertaken in the United States—will help determine, among other things, the risks of long-term hormone therapy to the heart and bones.

What's a woman to do in the meantime? Working with your physician, weigh the benefits and risks of long-term hormone use, factoring in your family history of heart disease, osteoporosis, and cancer, as well as risk factors such as smoking, cholesterol levels, and bone density. Knowledge is your best ally.

To find out if you are a candidate for HRT, look at the risk/benefit analysis below and check off the risk factors that apply to you. If you are at high risk of heart disease and osteoporosis, you should consider hormone replacement therapy. If you are at high risk of osteoporosis, the medication Fosamax, or other bisphosphonates such as Didrocal and Actonel, should be considered if you don't want to use HRT. If you are at risk for breast cancer and fear that HRT will increase that risk, continue with your monthly self-examination and periodic mammograms.

Check Your Risk Factors

Women considering hormone replacement therapy should consider the following risk factors when making their decision.

Heart Disease Risks

- You have had a heart attack.
- One of your parents suffered a heart attack before the age of fifty-five.
- Your cholesterol level is over 240 and you have HDL below 30, LDL above 160, and triglycerides above 200.
- You have diabetes.
- You smoke.
- You are not physically active.
- You are more than 30 percent over the ideal weight for your height and age.
- Your blood pressure is high (above 140/90).
- You reached menopause before age forty.

Osteoporosis Risks

- You are Caucasian or Asian.
- You are a thin woman with a small-boned frame and fair hair.
- You have a family history of osteoporosis.
- You are not physically active.
- You have a low intake of calcium (less than 1,500 mg daily).
- You smoke.
- You drink excessively—more than 2 drinks daily (a drink is defined as 5 ounces of wine, 1.5 ounces of 80-proof liquor, or 12 ounces of beer).

- You reached menopause before age forty.
- You have hyperthyroidism or hypothyroidism.
- You have had surgery to remove your ovaries.
- You have had radiation treatment for ovarian cancer.
- You have used cortisone-based drugs for a long period of time.

Breast Cancer Risks

- You or your mother, sister, or daughter has had breast cancer.
- You have certain mutations of the BRCA (breast susceptibility) genes.
- You reached menopause after the age of fifty.
- You never had children.
- You gave birth after the age of thirty.
- You are physically inactive.
- You drink excessively (see above).

12

Balance Training Can Save Your Life

If exercise could be packed into a pill, it would be the most
widely prescribed—and beneficial—medicine in the nation.
—DR. ROBERT BUTLER

Imagine that you're an astronaut rocketing toward Mars. Glancing
around the spacecraft shortly after liftoff, you suddenly find your
nose inches from the ceiling, your legs floating up eerily behind you.
When you will your right leg to rise, it suddenly appears next to your
stomach, but once you relax, the leg disappears, exactly where you're
not quite sure.

Looking down—or at least you think it's down—you see the chair
you were previously strapped into. Closing your eyes for a moment,
you can no longer tell whether you're head up or down. With no pull
of gravity, your world has changed dramatically. Reference points
from Earth no longer work for you, and your brain starts spinning.

Sideways. Up. Down. You're no longer sure where you are. You become greatly confused and begin to feel sick.

The Visuo-Vestibular Mismatch

With the loss of gravity in space travel, the body's sense of balance is
short-circuited within ten minutes of liftoff. Microgravity quickly

takes its toll on the normal functioning of the vestibular apparatus in the inner ear. This is the fluid-filled network of canals deep within the ear that helps us keep our balance. In microgravity, otoconia (the microscopic calcium crystals) no longer bend the twenty thousand protruding fibers, called cilia, that help regulate balance. The body quickly loses its innate sense of where it is in space, and distinguishing up from down becomes a major problem.

When it comes to maintaining a sense of balance in space, muscle and bone no longer send meaningful signals, so visual cues take on a more important role. Your eyes can tell you that you're upside down but stable, but your brain—still working as if it were on Earth—insists that you're falling and in danger of hurting yourself. Such balance dysfunction frequently causes what's known as a *visuo-vestibular mismatch*, and when that happens, the brain becomes flustered.

The majority of American astronauts and Russian cosmonauts have experienced in-flight vestibular disorientation, including sensations of tumbling or rotation and vertigo. Your sense of balance depends on *proprioception*, which is the information your brain receives from your inner ear, your eyes, and the receptors in your muscles, tendons, and joints, which then tell the brain where your body— spine, neck, arms, ankles, hips, and shoulders—is in space. Without the familiar stresses in the joints usually caused by the pull of gravity, the nerves in the body's joints and muscles that tell us where our arms and legs are in space are fooled. The end result is space sickness: nausea and vomiting that can last for several days.

NASA researchers believe that space sickness is much like the motion sickness people develop when they try to read in a moving car. While the inner ear detects the motion of the moving car, the eyes, staring at the page, do not. The conflicting information, sent rapid-fire to the brain from the eyes and inner ear, results in the all-too-familiar cold sweats, nausea, and vomiting.

Astronauts afflicted with space sickness soon get over the ailment, typically within seventy-two hours of liftoff. The nausea stops as the brain begins to readapt, coming to trust the eyes and starting to reprogram signals to the vestibular system to fix any of the mismatches it is now receiving.

NASA researchers are still at work trying to solve this vexing balance problem for the astronauts, searching for ways not only to prevent and treat space sickness but also to help astronauts quickly regain their balance when they come back from their mission in space.

A Sense of Where You Are

A sense of balance, which I liken to a "sixth sense," is a complex ability we develop when we're young and then take for granted—until we have balance problems. As young children, we learned to sit, crawl, walk, and then run. At a young age we learned to ride a bike, ice skate, ski, dance, dive, do somersaults, and elude tacklers on a football field. To do so, myriad complex messages were continually sent to the brain from the body's various balance sensors. What we've done over time is learn how to translate all of the sensory information picked up from various systems—nerves, muscles, bone, and eyes—and use it so we can move with grace.

When you are strong, a push to the chest or back alerts the ankle joints to send a message to the brain to stimulate the calf muscles to resist the shove and steady the ankles and feet. Once these muscles go into action, the body is on its way to becoming centered and balance is quickly restored.

As the years pass and we use our muscles less and less, the sedentary lifestyle weakens the body dramatically and the sensory information sent to the brain becomes muddled or even ceases. The end result is that you gradually begin to lose your balance. You're no longer as steady on your feet as before. This becomes apparent when you play sports and you struggle to perform as you once did, or when you try to reach for some canned goods stored high up on your pantry shelf and find yourself worried about falling off the chair.

One in three people sixty-five and older falls, mainly due to lack of balance. Physical inactivity is the culprit. Decreased muscle size and strength greatly reduce coordination and reaction time. Some physically frail people are so afraid of falling that their apprehension may actually increase their risk of falling. When a person is afraid a fall will occur, he or she assumes safer postures by standing with feet far- ther apart and walking with slower, smaller steps. Although these ad- justments are made to maintain balance, they actually contribute to decreased sensory input, decreased mobility, and an increased loss of flexibility and strength that unfortunately leads to falls.

Balance Training Has No Age Limits

Before beginning my strength-training studies, I often ask volun- teers to try the one-leg balance test. I have them stand close to a sturdy chair that they can grab, if need be, close their eyes, and then raise one knee. Younger people have no problem with this and can usually hold the position for at least thirty seconds before they lose their balance. Those older than forty often find the exercise to be dif- ficult, with many losing their balance and putting their foot down in less than fifteen seconds. Those past sixty often cannot make it longer than ten seconds.

The good news is that balance, just like strength and endurance, can be preserved and developed. The gradual loss of hair cells deep within the inner ear is inevitable, but weak muscles are not. When you keep your muscles, you maintain the important strength that's so essential for balance.

Balance is critical in everyday activities, but it's something that's rarely worked on by anyone. We all have the ability to make sig- nificant improvements in our balance, however, which can lead to greater coordination, improved posture and stability, and enhanced athletic performance.

E-Centrics, combined with the AstroFit balance exercises, have kept me strong and agile like a cat. And if I do stumble, I find that I'm able to right myself more readily than ever before.

—*Rosalie*

Testing Your Balance

Balance training, the missing element in most conditioning programs, is all about developing and enhancing better communication between the brain and the body's muscles. To determine your current level of balance, try these simple tests right now.

The Up-and-Go Test

This simple test evaluates your current balance status. You will need someone with a watch to time you.

Wearing regular footwear, get up out of a standard armchair (with a seat height of eighteen inches), walk ten feet as quickly as you can, turn, walk back to the chair, and sit down. If this takes thirty seconds or more, it means you have impaired strength, mobility, and balance and are at high risk of falling.

Balance Test

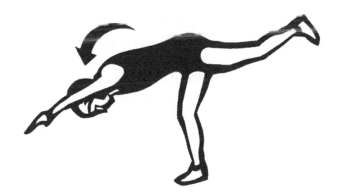

- Stand on one foot with the other foot slightly raised and behind you.
- Reach forward and touch the floor in front of you and then stand up straight again—all the time balanced on one foot.
- Switch feet and repeat the exercise.

Don't be surprised if you find yourself swaying from side to side, with your arms flailing, as you try to stay balanced on one foot. The good news is that with regular practice, you'll soon be able to perform this exercise with ease.

Balance Training

Having good balance means that you unconsciously know where your center of gravity is so you can position yourself to sit, walk, run, throw, kick, or push. If you want to improve your balance, you need to work on enhancing it. For most people, even a highly trained athlete or dedicated exerciser, these seemingly simple balance exercises often prove to be quite difficult at first.

Balance training forces you to use a variety of muscles that stabilize your body. These include the muscles of your feet, ankles, and calves, but more specifically those in your core. The core area, also known as "the power zone," is where your center of gravity is located. It's made up of the muscles, tendons, ligaments and connective tissue from the lower chest to just below your navel, and in your back from your neck to your buttocks. Strengthening the core improves your posture, with the strong abdominals holding your whole body up, keeping it centered over your feet.

No matter what your fitness level, you can now greatly improve your balance with a variety of exercises that make use of your eyes, feet, and inner ear. These balance exercises can be performed at home, without any elaborate equipment. An eight-foot piece of rope is enough to add a challenging level of difficulty to ordinary movements, postures, and exercises.

When performed at least once a week, these exercises will enhance your coordination, body awareness, and control, and also help prevent injuries. Keep at it. The next time you slip but are able to avoid falling, you'll realize the value of the balance exercises.

Balance Workout Guidelines

The following exercises will challenge your balance by displacing your legs and hips in as many controlled actions as possible. In addition to training your brain to monitor movement through receptors in your muscles, tendons, joints, and skin, these exercises will also help strengthen the muscles in your feet and lower leg as you try to maintain balance.

With some practice, your balance awareness will improve dramatically, and in a short while you may find yourself breezing through much of what had once been a challenging routine.

There are two progressive phases to the AstroFit balance program. Begin with Phase One, with five exercises. One balance session per week is sufficient. Once you are able to complete the exercises with relative ease, I hope you will move on to Phase Two and its five more challenging exercises.

Phase One Balance Training

1. Hip flexion
2. Side leg raise
3. Toe raises
4. Knee flexion
5. Heel-to-toe walking

EXERCISE 1: HIP FLEXION

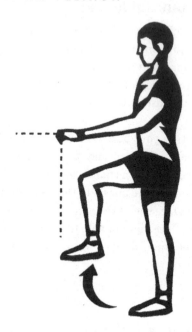

Get Set

- Stand straight, holding on to a table or chair with your hand for balance.

The Movement

- Slowly bend one knee toward your chest, without bending at your waist or hips.
- Hold this position for thirty seconds.
- Slowly lower the leg back to the starting position.
- Repeat with the other leg.

Note: As you progress and this becomes too easy, try the same exercise while holding on with one fingertip; without holding on to anything; and finally, with your eyes closed. When exercising with your eyes closed, you may struggle at first, which goes to show how much you rely on your eyesight to maintain equilibrium. Again, with practice your muscles will take over for your eyes and maintain the body in proper equilibrium.

EXERCISE 2: SIDE LEG RAISE

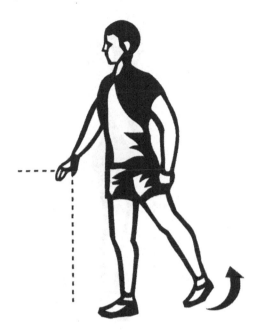

Get Set
- Stand straight, directly behind a table or chair, feet slightly apart.
- Hold on with one hand for balance.

The Movement
- Keeping your knees and leg straight, slowly lift one leg to the side, six to twelve inches.
- Hold the position for thirty seconds.
- Slowly lower the leg back to the starting position.
- Repeat with your other leg.

Note: As you progress and this becomes too easy, try the same exercise while holding on with one fingertip; without holding on to anything; and finally, with your eyes closed.

EXERCISE 3: TOE RAISES

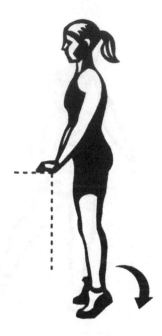

Get Set

- Stand straight, holding on to a table or chair with your hand for balance.

The Movement

- Slowly raise yourself up on tiptoe as high as possible.
- Hold the position for five seconds.
- Slowly lower your heels to the starting position.
- Repeat fifteen times. Rest a minute and repeat.

Note: As you progress and this becomes too easy, try the same exercise while holding on with one fingertip; without holding on to anything; and finally, with your eyes closed.

EXERCISE 4: KNEE FLEXION

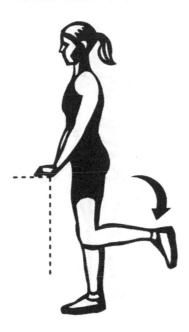

Get Set

- Stand straight, holding on to a table or chair with your hand for balance.

The Movement

- Slowly bend your knee as far as possible, so your foot lifts up behind you.
- Hold the position for thirty seconds.
- Slowly lower your foot all the way back down.
- Repeat with your other leg.

Note: As you progress and this becomes too easy, try the same exercise while holding on with one fingertip; without holding on to anything; and finally, with your eyes closed.

EXERCISE 5: HEEL-TO-TOE WALKING

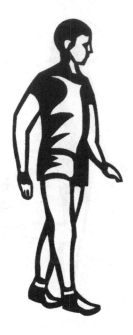

Get Set

- Position your heel just in front of the toes of the opposite foot. Your heel and toes should touch or almost touch.

The Movement

- Start walking, with your heels and toes touching or almost touching.
- Walk forward twenty feet, turn around, and walk back to the starting position.

Note: As you progress and this becomes too easy, try the same exercise but walk *backward*.

Phase Two Balance Training

1. Knee lifts
2. Stair steppers

3. Hop-alongs
4. Balance walking
5. One-legged squats

EXERCISE 1: KNEE LIFTS

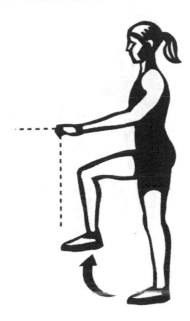

Get Set
- Stand straight with your feet shoulder width apart, holding on to
  a table or chair with your hand for support.
The Movement
- Lift your left knee up to hip level and hold for thirty seconds.
- Return to the starting position, stand on your left foot, and
  repeat the exercise.

Note: For an extra challenge, have a partner gently push you with
his or her fingertips from various angles, trying to make you sway.

EXERCISE 2: STAIR STEPPERS

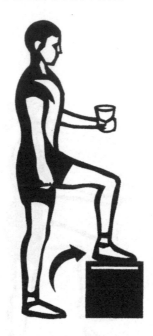

Get Set

- Stand in front of a low step, holding a full cup of water in both hands.

The Movement

- Step up as quickly as you can, first with your right foot and then your left.
- Step down with your right foot and then with your left without spilling the water.
- Repeat five times.

EXERCISE 3: HOP-ALONGS

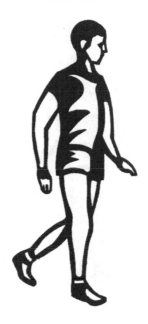

Get Set

- Balance on your right foot.

The Movement

- Hop forward four times.
- Hop backward four times.
- Switch to your left foot and repeat.

EXERCISE 4: BALANCE WALKING

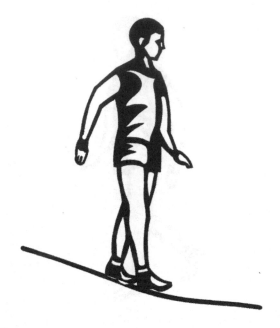

Get Set
- Place an eight-foot piece of rope in a straight line on the floor.
The Movement
- Walk on the rope as if it were a tightrope suspended above the ground.
- When you reach the end of the rope, slowly turn around and return to the start.
- When that becomes easy, complete the drill by tossing a tennis ball from one hand to the other as you walk.

EXERCISE 5: ONE-LEGGED SQUATS

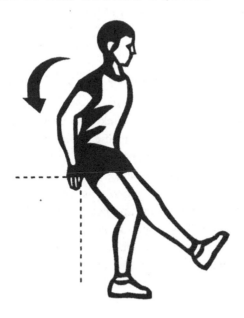

Get Set

- Holding on to a table or chair for support, stand on your right foot, with your left foot either behind or in front of you.

The Movement

- Slowly bend your right knee, keeping your foot flat on the floor as your buttocks move backward.
- Keep your right kneecap aligned over and between your first and second toes.
- Continue to lower your body until your upper thigh is almost parallel to the floor.
- Pause momentarily.
- Push upward forcefully with your quadriceps to the starting position.

Note: For increasing levels of difficulty, your hands can be held out to the sides, on your hips, or across your chest. You can take the intensity up another notch by tossing a tennis ball with one hand while performing the movement. Once this becomes relatively simple, try performing the exercise standing on a seat cushion. This less stable base of support will provide a greater challenge.

Injecting Balance Drills into Daily Activities

In addition to these ten specific balance exercises, I also incorporate many of my daily activities into a makeshift balance program. For example, every time I find myself waiting in line at the supermarket, or when I'm standing at the sink brushing my teeth, I lift one of my feet up a few inches and stand on one leg. I alternate my feet every thirty seconds—or when I lose my balance, whichever comes first.

For the more adventuresome and coordinated: If you are standing in a moving vehicle (bus, train, subway), try standing on one foot while holding lightly on to a support bar to prevent a fall. If this isn't challenging enough, close your eyes and stand on one foot.

This type of training may not be at the top of your list of important things to accomplish. However, in years to come, when you're still lithe and physically active and able to move with grace, power, and confidence, I can guarantee you'll be glad you took the time.

Five

Optimal Nutrition

13

Fuel Your Muscles

A strong body makes the mind strong.
—THOMAS JEFFERSON

On the trip to Mars, I want the astronauts to maintain their muscles in order to stave off the aging that would otherwise occur on their voyage. In addition to regular strength training—the high-intensity E-Centric strength-building program—this will be accomplished by carefully planned meals.

My Mars-designed AstroFit program is also critically important for us on Earth. My research has already demonstrated that once we gain maturity (at about age twenty-five for men and seventeen or eighteen for women), we start to lose muscle and bone. Not only does this loss affect our strength and stamina, it also affects our daily caloric requirement. Our metabolic rate decreases in direct proportion to the amount of muscle lost. Most of us do not change our diets as we age, so as we continue to eat the same way, we gain fat. The body of an average twenty-year-old man is about 18 percent fat, skyrocketing to 38 percent fat by age sixty. For a woman, the pattern is similar but the numbers are even more pronounced: the average twenty-year-old woman is about 23 percent fat; forty years later, she's 44 percent fat.

It's important for all of us to realize that we don't just wake up one day and discover that we have lost muscle and gained fat.

This is a lifelong, gradual process. But it's one that doesn't have to happen.

Making Wise Food Choices

Over the years, I've encountered many people who exercise regularly, only to have their efforts undermined by what they eat. When you exercise, you need to consume more protein, especially right after E-Centric workouts, when the muscles begin their repair-and-rebuilding process. You also need other macronutrients—water, carbohydrate, fat, and protein—in your diet to optimize muscle growth. And you need to time your meals correctly so the food you consume is put to the best use.

Making wise food choices and eating at the precisely correct time is just as important to your success in AstroFit as performing the E-Centrics correctly. *What* you eat and *when* you eat it will go a long way to keeping you energetic, fueling your body, and priming it to build lean body tissue while paring away excess body fat.

To make it easier for you, I've provided fourteen days' worth of delicious AstroFit meal choices in the next chapter, in addition to fifty-four recipes. Each hearty meal is based on my 60-20-20 eating plan, with 60 percent of the nutrients coming from carbohydrates, 20 percent from protein, and the remaining 20 percent from fats. This plan is not about limiting food, but rather eating plenty of nutritious foods throughout the course of the day. In addition to building lean muscle mass, this frequent eating will keep you from feeling overly hungry and then consuming an enormous meal at the end of the day—the habit of too many Americans.

By eating smaller quantities of food every two to three hours, you will keep your insulin levels fairly stable. Insulin is the hormone that regulates your muscles' uptake of nutrients and calories. Steady levels of insulin mean that calories are more easily converted to the glycogen that is used to fuel muscle activity. The AstroFit diet decreases the risk of diabetes (an epidemic in the United States) and heart disease. Because the diet is rich in carbohydrates, it promotes insulin production and therefore stimulates protein synthesis and limits muscle protein breakdown.

Adhering to the various eating suggestions will not guarantee that you will be able to set records in how much weight you can lift in twelve weeks or that you'll be able to run faster and farther, but this balanced nutritional approach is certain to help you optimize your workouts. The food choices that I recommend provide energy, support new muscle repair and growth, and assist in regulating your metabolism. With countless test subjects having already achieved success on the AstroFit nutrition plan, I can assure you that it works very well.

Over the past decade, I have tried just about every diet ever invented—and failed with them all. Not only did I lose weight with the AstroFit plan and keep it off for two years, but I have well-defined muscles and I'm much more alert and have more energy than I ever had in my life.

—*Barbara, age 44*

The 60-20-20 Plan

My formula for fueling your muscles is easy to follow. Each day, you should consume approximately 60 percent of your total calories from carbohydrate, 20 percent from protein, and 20 percent from fat. The beauty of this eating ratio is that it is ideal for maximum muscle growth and can be continued for a lifetime of healthful eating.

It's important to note that what's considered adequate nutrition for the nonexerciser is most likely not adequate to meet your body's requirements. A person following the AstroFit program has increased energy needs and must consume more of the energy-yielding macronutrients in the right proportions.

I am currently conducting an extensive study sponsored by the National Institutes of Health to examine the effects of the AstroFit diet. Our preliminary results demonstrate that consuming such a diet *ad libitum* (in other words, eating as much as you desire with no specific restrictions on calorie consumption) produces significant weight loss. The number of calories you consume is not as important as keeping the 60-20-20 ratio. While many new dietary regimens recommend the elimination of carbohydrates, our research has demonstrated that carbohydrate consumption increases your BMR (the number of calories you burn at rest) and promotes muscle building as a result of the anabolic properties of insulin.

Eat Frequently

In addition to breakfast, lunch, and dinner, you will have a mid-morning, midafternoon, and pre-bed snack. It's been demonstrated that exercisers who eat throughout the day have significantly lower levels of body fat than those who eat three larger meals a day. This is because frequent meals even out your blood sugar so that you don't have the peaks and valleys that cause your body to defend its fat supply. And since your body doesn't store amino acids, the frequent meals ensure that these all-important building blocks of muscle are present when they are needed.

Carbohydrates: Your Primary Energy Source

Carbohydrates—sugars and starches, which are found in plant foods such as vegetables, grains, legumes, and fruits—are your most readily available source of nutrient energy. Perform an E-Centric squat or leg press, and it's carbohydrate that supplies almost 95 percent of the muscle fuel.

I liken carbs to the gasoline you put in your car. Through digestion and metabolism, all carbohydrate stored in the body is converted into *glucose,* a blood sugar that flows through the bloodstream and is "burned" as one source of fuel for the body and the only source of energy for the brain. Glucose that is not used to provide energy is transported by the blood to your liver and muscle tissues, where it is stored until needed as a substance called *glycogen.*

Simple carbohydrates (commonly known as sugars), are found mainly in fruits and milk. *Complex carbohydrates* (commonly known as starches), such as whole grains, bread, pasta, cereal, rice, potatoes, and legumes, help maintain your muscle glycogen. The hormone *insulin,* which is released from the pancreas, facilitates the transport of glucose from the blood to the sites of glycogen storage. Insulin also helps prevent the breakdown of protein for energy.

Your Carbohydrate Requirement

In the AstroFit plan, I use the ratio of 60-20-20. While the AstroFit plan has no restriction on total calorie intake, 60 percent of your daily calories will come from carbohydrate sources.

Most of us have only a vague idea of how many calories we should consume daily. Typically, we just eat until we are no longer hungry. Here is a better way to estimate your carbohydrate needs.

First, you must calculate your approximate resting metabolic rate. As you recall from Chapter 5, your resting metabolic rate is largely determined by your fat-free body mass. The following formula for determining fat-free mass takes into account weight, gender, and age, each of which contributes to the total amount of fat-free mass that you have.

Formula to Determine Resting Energy Expenditure

Men:

18–30 years old	(15.3 × weight in kilograms) + 679
30–60	(11.6 × weight in kilograms) + 879
60+	(13.5 × weight in kilograms) + 487

Women:

18–30	(14.7 × weight in kilograms) + 496
30–60	(8.7 × weight in kilograms) + 829
60+	(10.5 × weight in kilograms) + 596

Source: National Research Council, *Recommended Dietary Allowances,* 10th ed. (Washington, D.C.: National Academy Press, 1989), p. 26.

In this formula, weight is expressed in kilograms. To convert your weight in pounds to kilograms, simply divide by 2.2.

Let's use the example of John, a forty-five-year-old man who weighs 190 pounds.

1. $(11.6 \times \frac{190}{2.2}) + 879 = 1{,}002 + 879 = 1{,}881 =$ resting energy expenditure (REE) in calories per day
2. 1,881 calories per day is John's resting metabolic rate, or his approximate energy expenditure. (This is how many calories he burns up if he just stays in bed and doesn't use his muscles for any physical activity.)

Since we are physical beings and not bedridden, we also have to determine the activity factor. In my research, I have calculated this to be 1.7 times your REE for people under the age of sixty and 1.6 times your REE for people over sixty.

Using John again as our example, here's how to figure his total daily energy needs:

1,881 calories per day × 1.7 = 3,198 calories per day

This is the approximate number of calories John will need to provide the energy for his daily activities.

Once we know John's approximate daily caloric requirements, it's a simple process to determine his carbohydrate allotment. Since 60 percent of these calories should come from carbohydrates, let's take a look at the numbers to determine the daily calories and grams from carbohydrates.

1. 3,198 calories per day × 0.6 = 1,919 calories per day from carbohydrates.
2. Each gram of carbohydrate contains 4 calories: $\frac{1919}{4}$ calories per gram = 480 grams of carbohydrate per day. This is the number of grams of carbohydrate that John should consume daily.

The Problem with Low-Carbohydrate Diets

Carbohydrate-limited diets produce significant weight loss. The weight is lost for two reasons:

- All carbohydrates are stored as glycogen in the liver and muscles. Once you restrict the carbohydrates you consume, you quickly start using up your body stores of carbohydrate, particularly those in the liver. All of the glycogen in the liver can be depleted in two to three days on a very-low-carbohydrate diet.
- *Diuresis,* or excessive urination, begins. Water is stored along with carbohydrate, so that as you use up your glycogen, the water is released. If you weigh yourself frequently, you become pleasantly surprised that you are losing a lot of weight within the first week of going on the low-carb diet. However, this is not fat that's being lost but water weight.

Once you go off the low-carbohydrate diet and increase your carbohydrate intake, glycogen and water storage increases rapidly, resulting in a *large* increase in weight. More than 95 percent of those who have lost a significant amount of weight on low-carbohydrate diets have gained it all back within one year.

Fat Basics

Fats, or lipids (the Greek word for "fat" is *lipos*), commonly contribute as many as 45 percent of the calories in the typical American diet, a level far higher than necessary to maintain optimal health. Fats are a natural component of some foods (such as whole milk, meat, nuts, and cheese), and they are often added in food processing (to make, for example, potato chips and desserts).

Fat is a concentrated source of energy, providing more than twice the potential energy of protein or carbohydrate. To maintain good health, your diet must contain adequate amounts of fat sources that supply essential fatty acids. Essential fatty acids play a vital role in energy production, stabilizing blood sugar, balancing hormones, and controlling hunger.

Good fat sources are those that are unprocessed and occur naturally in foods. High-quality fat sources include olive oil, fish and fish oils, vegetable oils, and all types of raw nuts and seeds.

Your Fat Requirements

In the AstroFit plan, 20 percent of your daily calories will come from fat. Here's the two-step process to determine your fat needs. Using the same example of John, the 190-pound, forty-five-year-old man we visited in the carbohydrate section, here's how to figure out your daily fat needs.

We know that John should consume 3,198 calories per day. Since 20 percent of these calories should come from fat, here are the numbers:

1. 3,198 calories per day × 0.2 = 640 calories per day from fat.
2. Fat is more calorie-laden than carbohydrate or protein. Each gram of fat contains 9 calories: $\frac{640}{9}$ calories per gram = 71 grams of fat. This is the number of grams of fat that John should consume daily.

Protein: The Misunderstood Macronutrient

The word protein comes from the Greek word *proteios*, which means "of primary importance." This is a fitting word since protein is a major component of hormones, antibodies, enzymes, and tissues, accounts for about 20 percent of your weight, and is essential in the repair of cells, including muscle cells. Many bodybuilders and some daily exercisers believe they can never get enough protein. Distance runners generally don't get enough, but the average American consumes far too much protein—and fat—than is necessary for good health.

My research shows that people following the AstroFit plan need to consume 250 percent more than the Recommended Dietary Allowance (RDA) for protein—and they need to have some protein with every meal. Because protein is an essential component of muscle structure, consuming a sufficient amount after exercise ensures proper repair and development of your muscle cells.

Protein is synthesized by the body from *amino acids,* the primary building blocks of protein. The body combines the amino acids it needs to build muscle. Of the many amino acids that your body uses to make protein, eleven are called *nonessential amino acids* because they can be produced by your body from other amino acids and do not need to be obtained from your diet. However, your body cannot make nine essential amino acids. They come from animals and include meat, eggs, fish, poultry, and milk and dairy products. These food products are called *complete proteins* because they contain all nine essential amino acids that must be present in order for your body to build or repair muscle.

The digestive system breaks all proteins down into their amino acids so that they can enter the bloodstream. Cells then use the amino acids as building blocks. In order for the body to synthesize lean tissue, all the essential amino acids must be available simultaneously. A nonessential amino acid that is in short supply can be produced by the liver. However, if even one essential amino acid is missing, the body must break down tissue—such as muscle—to obtain it.

To prevent muscle cell breakdown, the dietary protein you consume daily must supply all the essential amino acids. While carbohydrates can be stored in the muscle and liver as glycogen, there is only a small amino acid pool in the bloodstream. To maintain the *optimal* environment for muscle growth (positive nitrogen balance) complete proteins must be eaten with every meal.

Essential Amino Acids

Histidine	Phenylalanine
Isoleucine	Threonine
Leucine	Tryptophan
Lysine	Valine
Methionine	

Nonessential Amino Acids

Alanine	Glutamine
Arginine	Glycine
Asparagine	Proline
Aspartic acid	Serine
Cysteine	Tryosine
Glutamic acid	

Animal Protein Sources

Since an animal's body is similar to our own, animal protein sources contain all the essential amino acids. Consume two four-ounce servings of animal protein—what we call "high-quality protein"—and you're almost assured of meeting your minimum daily needs. See the chart on page 228 for a more detailed list of protein sources.

Vegetable Protein Sources

Except for soybeans, vegetable protein sources are usually low in certain essential amino acids or missing them altogether. Many grains lack the amino acids lysine and threonine, while beans lack methionine, so vegetarians, especially vegans, may be at risk of developing protein deficiency. However, the body can make complete proteins when a variety of plant foods—vegetables, fruits, beans, grains, nuts, and seeds—and sufficient calories are consumed during the day. A half cup of cooked whole-grain pasta (3 grams of protein), a cup of cooked beans (12 grams), an ounce of nuts (5 grams), and a tablespoon of peanut butter (4 grams) are all examples of plant-based proteins that will help meet your protein needs. Just remember that some protein sources contain more fat than others.

Eggs

One of the best sources of high-quality protein is eggs. Not only do eggs contain all of the essential amino acids, but they're also a rich source of folic acid, vitamins B_{12}, E, and D, as well as thiamine, riboflavin, and pantothenic acid. More than half the egg's protein is in the white, while all of the fat is in the yolk.

For years, health-conscious exercisers have been scared away from eggs due to their high cholesterol content (210 milligrams). However, recent medical research now indicates that consuming an egg daily does not increase your risk of coronary heart disease and that consuming two eggs a day shouldn't make any difference if you generally follow a low-fat eating program such as the AstroFit plan.

Eggs' Nutritional Breakdown

1 large egg white: 17 calories, 3.5 g protein, 0.3 g carbohydrate, 0 g fat

1 large whole egg: 77 calories, 6.3 g protein, 0.6 g carbohydrate, 5 g fat

Protein as a Muscle Fuel

For years, my research has focused on how the body uses protein, with a particular focus on its effects on exercise and aging. For the longest time, it was assumed that exercise had very little—if any—

effect on the need for protein. Most nutrition and exercise scientists believed that the only fuels needed for muscles were carbohydrates and fats. However, studies carried out in my lab, and the labs of other researchers, have demonstrated that we do use protein as a fuel during workouts.

I determined this by placing a catheter into the veins of volunteers and then infusing the amino acid leucine, along with an isotope label so it could be tracked. While the test subjects were exercising on a treadmill, I examined the air they were exhaling. The amount of carbon dioxide that contained the isotope alerted me to how much leucine the runners were actually burning as a fuel.

As I suspected, the use of leucine was significant. The use of protein as fuel was a relatively small percentage of the total energy demand of the exercise—only about 7 percent of all of the fuel during the exercise came from protein. Still, it was clear that the body's requirement of protein must be greater in those who engage in regular aerobic exercise.

To answer the question of whether or not increased consumption of protein is important in the muscle-building response to resistance training, I conducted another metabolic balance study. For this study, healthy but previously sedentary men and women were recruited. Half of these subjects consumed the RDA of 0.8 gram of protein per kilogram of body weight, while the remaining subjects consumed double this amount—1.6 grams of protein. All other aspects of their diets remained the same. These volunteers were then put through a three-day-per-week resistance-training program for three months.

The diets of the volunteers were strictly regulated, and we prevented them from gaining or losing weight. Everyone was weighed daily, and if a person lost weight, we increased his or her food intake. Portions were cut if weight was gained. In this way, we could determine exactly how many calories each of the research subjects required to maintain his or her body weight.

After three months of performing the prescribed program of resistance exercise three days per week, we found that the men and women had to consume an average of almost 15 percent more food than when they had entered the study—almost 400 calories extra each day! Many of the volunteers admitted that as they had gotten stronger, they had become more active. They walked more, climbed stairs, and began doing more physical activities throughout the day. This accounted for some of the caloric increase. The major reason for their increased caloric boost, however, came from the fact that weight training caused them to "rev up their engines" and begin burning more calories. Weight training and its ongoing muscle building required more calories, and the increased muscle mass had its own caloric demands.

Unlike aerobic exercise, which causes an increase in caloric consumption for up to a few hours after the activity is over, weight-training sessions cause calories to be burned twenty-four hours a day. Interestingly, we also found that those who consumed the high-protein diet gained 5 to 10 percent more muscle than those consuming the RDA for protein. This provided ample evidence that the amount of dietary protein intake can influence how much muscle is gained from strength training.

After a hard workout, your body calls for more amino acids and proteins. If you're serious about this program, you will need between 0.5 gram and 1 gram of protein per pound of body weight each day. That's about a minimum of 85 grams of protein daily for a 170-pound E-Centric exerciser, or about 250 percent of the current Recommended Dietary Allowance of 0.36 gram per pound for nonexercising, sedentary adults. As you continue training over the weeks, your body adapts to the E-Centric stress by synthesizing more protein in each muscle cell. This process causes the muscles to become larger so they can handle heavier weights. With more muscle, you'll soon find that the fifteen- or twenty-pound dumbbell that was once hard to lift offers no challenge whatsoever four or five weeks later.

Calculate Your Protein Requirements

Be aware that in trying to ensure adequate protein intake, you need to consume just the right amount to minimize the formation of metabolic waste products. When too much protein is consumed, the body converts the excess to fat, which then increases the blood levels of ammonia and uric acid. These are toxic metabolic waste products. Therefore your goal is to maintain a proper, balanced protein intake. You can determine your approximate protein requirements with the following formula.

Multiply your weight in pounds by the minimum number of grams of protein (0.5), and then by the maximum number of grams of protein (1.0).

Example: Janet weighs 150 pounds, so the formula would work out like this:

To determine her minimum daily protein needs:
Multiply weight in pounds by 0.5 gram
150 × 0.5 gram = 75 grams per day
To determine her maximum daily protein needs:
Multiply weight in pounds by 1.0 gram
150 × 1.0 gram per kilogram = 150 grams per day

Protein Supplements

You can't walk into a supermarket, grocery store, or health food store these days without seeing canisters of protein powders and protein meal replacements and stacks of protein bars on the shelves. Should you incorporate them into your AstroFit plan? That all depends on your particular needs. You could benefit from the additional protein if you are looking for a convenient pre- and postworkout snack (or meal option), if you're a vegetarian and need to meet your daily protein needs, or if you have had a particularly hard workout and want a quick protein-rich snack.

Whey Protein

Whey, a dairy-based source of high-quality amino acids that was once thought to be a worthless by-product of cheese production, has recently become one of the most popular protein supplements—and with good reason. Whey protein has the highest levels of branched-chain amino acids—leucine, isoleucine, and valine—of any single protein source. These are the first amino acids used by the body during an intense E-Centric session.

Another benefit of whey is its fast absorption rate. Whey protein exits the stomach much faster than other proteins and is absorbed more quickly into the bloodstream through the intestines. This is important during exercise as well as recovery.

Finally, whey protein enhances the production of glutathione. Glutathione is one of the body's most powerful natural antioxidants. While you are exercising, the extra glutathione is at work protecting against cellular free-radical damage caused by the workout. Free radicals are minute entities that are produced by the body in response to the cell's natural process of using oxygen for metabolism. The free radicals can harm basic genetic material, cell walls, and other cell structures. The affected cells are then unable to perform their molecular work effectively, and in the long run this damage can become irreparable. Free-radical damage has been directly linked to heart disease and some types of cancer.

Several different methods are used to evaluate protein quality. Three methods are the Protein Digestibility—Corrected Amino Acid Score (PDCAAS), the Protein Efficiency Ratio (PER), and the Biological Value (BV). No matter which method is used, whey proteins have been proven to be an excellent, pure source of protein.

Soy Protein

Soybeans are packed with protein, offering all the benefits of protein found in meat, milk, and eggs but without the cholesterol and with less saturated fat. Not only does the soybean contain more protein than any other plant, but the protein it contains is of higher quality. Researchers have speculated for some time that the high soy intake in most Asian countries is somehow related to the corresponding low levels of heart disease and breast and prostate cancers.

Soybeans contain all nine of the essential amino acids needed by

Protein Quality Comparison

PROTEIN TYPE	PROTEIN DIGESTIBILITY—CORRECTED AMINO ACID SCORE (PDCAAS)(1)	PROTEIN EFFICIENCY RATIO (PER)(2)	BIOLOGICAL VALUE (BV)
Whey protein	1.00	3.2	100
Whole egg	1.00	3.8	88–100
Casein	1.00	2.5	80
Soy protein concentrate	0.99	2.2	74
Beef protein	0.92	2.9	80
Canned kidney beans	0.68	NA*	49†
Canned lentils	0.52	NA*	NA*
Wheat gluten	0.25	NA*	54

*Information not readily available.
†Value is for beans in general.
Sources: (1) Joint FAO/WHO Consultation, *Protein Quality Evaluation* (Rome: FAO, 1990); (2) FAO Nutrition Studies No. 24: *Amino Acid Content of Foods and Biological Data on Protein* (Rome: FAO, 1970); (3) Ibid.

the body, and they're in the right balance to meet the demands of anyone following the AstroFit eating plan. Soy protein also has powerful antioxidant benefits. Since soy has naturally occurring isoflavones—plant estrogens—it can help reduce muscle soreness and speed up your recovery from your workout. Soy comes in many forms, including fresh, canned, and frozen soybeans; dried raw soybeans; soy protein powder; soy nuts; soy milk; tofu; tempeh; miso; and meat substitutes.

Protein Pointers

The cornerstone of the AstroFit nutrition plan is adequate consumption of complete proteins. Here are some guidelines to remember:

* Space your protein intake so that you consume small amounts of protein throughout the day at every meal and snack. This en-

courages better blood sugar balance, improved weight control, and increased energy.

- For your protein sources, choose unprocessed meats, poultry, legumes (beans and lentils), whey powder, fish, and soy products (soy milk, tofu, miso, cooked soybeans, and soy powder).
- If you're a vegetarian, be sure to consume a wide variety of plant protein sources such as whole grains, legumes, seeds, and nuts. Stay away from nutrient-poor carbohydrates, such as white bread and white pasta and noodles.

Top Protein Sources

MEAT, FISH, AND POULTRY

In this table, the servings are all roughly equivalent in total calories, *not* in serving size. You'll see that 140 calories can "buy" you either 4 ounces of tuna (with 30 grams of protein and 2 grams of fat) or 2 ounces of steak (with 15 grams of protein and 9 grams of fat).

SERVING SIZE	FOOD	CALORIES	PROTEIN (GRAMS)	CARBOHYDRATE (GRAMS)	FAT (GRAMS)
4 ounces	Carp	114	20	0	6
4 ounces	Catfish	132	21	0	5
3 ounces	Chicken breast, baked	123	21	0	5
6 ounces	Clams	126	21	4	2
5 ounces	Haddock	123	26	0	1
3.5 ounces	Ham, deli	145	21	2	6
2 ounces	Lamb	125	15	0	7
6 ounces	Oysters	138	16	8	4
3 ounces	Salmon	121	16	0	5
5 ounces	Scallops	115	22	5	0
15	Shrimp	113	22	1	2
6 ounces	Sole	117	26	0	1
2 ounces	Steak	138	15	0	9
4 ounces	Tuna	140	30	0	2
2 ounces	Turkey breast	104	21	0	2

(continued on next page)

DAIRY PRODUCTS AND EGG

SERVING SIZE	FOOD	CALORIES	PROTEIN (GRAMS)	CARBOHYDRATE (GRAMS)	FAT (GRAMS)
1	Egg whites	117	4	Trace	0
1 cup	Milk, nonfat	86	8	12	Trace
8 ounces	Yogurt, nonfat	127	13	17	0

GRAINS

SERVING SIZE	FOOD	CALORIES	PROTEIN (GRAMS)	CARBOHYDRATE (GRAMS)	FAT (GRAMS)
1	Bagel	195	7	38	1
1 slice	Bread, whole wheat	61	2	11	1
1 ear	Corn on the cob	160	4	32	0
1 ounce	Cream of wheat	100	3	22	0
1	English muffin	127	5	25	1
1 ounce	Grape-Nuts	110	3	23	0
1 cup	Oatmeal	122	4	24	2
½ cup	Pasta	100	3	20	0
1 cup	Popcorn	54	2	11	1
1 cup	Rice, brown	216	5	45	2
1 cup	Rice, white	205	4	44	Trace
2	Rice cakes	70	1	16	0
½ cup	Shredded wheat	68	2	17	0
1 cup	Spaghetti	197	7	40	1
2 tablespoons	Wheat germ	50	4	6	1

VEGETABLES

SERVING SIZE	FOOD	CALORIES	PROTEIN (GRAMS)	CARBOHYDRATE (GRAMS)	FAT (GRAMS)
1 cup	Asparagus	44	5	8	1
1 ounce	Avocado	36	1	2	3
1 cup	Broccoli	46	5	9	0
2 cups	Cabbage	32	2	8	1
1	Carrot	31	1	7	0
6 stalks	Celery	36	2	9	1
2 cups	Cucumber	28	0	6	0
1 cup	Eggplant	26	1	6	0
1 cup	Kale	43	5	7	1
1 cup	Mushrooms	20	2	3	0
½ cup	Peas	59	4	11	0
1	Potato, baked	220	4	52	0
2 cups	Spinach	24	3	4	0

1 cup	Squash, summer	36	2	8	1
1	Tomato	34	2	8	0
½ cup	Tomato sauce	54	2	12	0

FRUITS, NUTS, AND LEGUMES

SERVING SIZE	FOOD	CALORIES	PROTEIN (GRAMS)	CARBOHYDRATE (GRAMS)	FAT (GRAMS)
1	Apple	80	0	24	0
3	Apricots	51	12	12	0
1	Banana	106	2	26	0
½ cup	Blueberries	41	1	10	0
½	Cantaloupe	94	2	22	11
½ cup	Cherries	52	1	12	1
3 ounces	Garbanzo beans	71	4	12	1
½	Grapefruit	41	1	11	0
½ cup	Grapes	57	1	11	0
1 cup	Lentils, cooked	300	18	40	0
1	Orange	62	1	15	0
1	Peach	38	1	10	1
2 tablespoons	Peanut butter	190	8	6	16
1 cup	Pineapple	77	1	19	1
1 cup	Raspberries	61	1	14	1
½ cup	Soybeans	149	14	9	8
1 cup	Strawberries	45	1	10	1
3.5 ounces	Tofu, firm	144	16	4	9
1 cup	Watermelon	59	1	12	0

Timing Is Everything

Protein is muscle food. When you begin E-Centric training, your muscles will be synthesizing a lot of new protein. However, without an adequate protein supply, the muscles you exercise may "borrow" protein from the muscles that are not being exercised. You don't want this to happen!

When you complete an E-Centric workout, your muscles are starving for amino acids to make new protein. The exercise has enhanced the sensitivity of your muscles to the hormone insulin. One of the many things insulin does is to stimulate muscle protein synthesis; it greatly increases the transport of amino acids from outside to inside the muscle cells that have been exercised.

This enhanced insulin sensitivity does not last for long. This means that if you want to help the muscle cells to make new protein, *you must consume the protein immediately after your workout,* along with some carbohydrate. The two macronutrients will work synergistically and stimulate insulin production. Insulin will cause muscles, particularly the ones you've been exercising, to "suck up" the amino acids like a sponge.

As you lift weights, the muscle cells are stimulated to increase the rate of muscle protein synthesis and breakdown. These cells are efficient in that the amino acids resulting from the breakdown of proteins are immediately reincorporated into newly synthesized protein. However, these cells need an abundance of amino acids—and not just any amino acids. They must include a complement of *all* of the essential amino acids.

The latest research shows that within thirty minutes after you complete E-Centric exercises is the ideal time to supply the nutrients for muscle cells with the necessary amino acids. In a recent study of elderly men who were put on a twelve-week resistance training program, gains of 22 percent were seen in muscle size when liquid protein was consumed right after the workouts. By comparison, men who consumed protein two hours after their workout bout showed no significant gain in muscle size.

The AstroBlast Protein Shake

I have found that during this time of increased transportation of amino acids into the muscles, the use of a protein supplement in liquid form will best maximize the gains that result from the workout. I have worked out a recipe for what I call the AstroBlast Protein Shake that you can make at home.

How much protein you use is based on how much you weigh. Typically, the amount of protein in one ounce of whey powder is about 20 grams. If you weigh between 100 and 150 pounds, use one ounce. If you weigh more than 150 pounds, use two ounces of the powder.

And don't forget chocolate flavoring. The two tablespoons of instant chocolate milk will add carbohydrate (sugar) to boost insulin production.

ASTROBLAST PROTEIN SHAKE

Makes 1 serving

3–5 ice cubes

2 tablespoons of instant chocolate milk

1 cup of soy milk or 1 percent milk

1–2 ounces of whey or soy protein powder

In a blender, combine all the ingredients. Process until the ice is all crushed and the drink is smooth. If the chocolate or protein powder sticks to the inside of the blender, use a spatula to scrape it off and blend for another ten seconds. Drink it all.

NUTRITION INFORMATION:
30 grams protein (with 1 ounce of powder and milk; 50 grams with 2 ounces of powder), 30 grams (approximately) carbohydrate

Marsha's Story

When I started to use AstroBlast with my test subjects, I began to see changes in their muscle growth patterns. Marsha is five feet seven and weighed 165 pounds with 27 percent body fat when I first saw her in my lab more than two years ago. I wanted her to alter her body composition so she had more muscle and less fat. This was okay with Marsha. She was consuming barely 1,200 calories a day and not losing weight. Her metabolism had been slowed down by low caloric intake, and she was holding on to more fat than she was burning.

The first thing we did was increase her meals from three to five per day, so she was now consuming close to 3,000 calories a day. She also began performing E-Centrics three times a week. She drank AstroBlast within thirty minutes after each workout.

Marsha's weight started dropping as her muscles began growing—

just as I had predicted. Marsha's body fat percentage is now 17, and she's a fit, energetic, healthy 134 pounds.

Marsha's case is not unique. When you change your way of eating and time your protein consumption to come right after your workout, beneficial results will occur.

Why AstroBlast Works

E-Centrics stimulate muscle growth. You stress the muscles, and they call out for protein and carbohydrate in order to rebuild and grow. Protein and carbohydrate stimulate the release of the hormone insulin. Insulin enhances the transport of amino acids into the cells, preventing muscle wasting and tissue loss. Insulin is what we call an "anabolic" hormone—it stimulates the building of protein. It is well known that simply increasing the percentage of calories from carbohydrates increases the efficiency of metabolizing protein, even without changing the amount of protein in the diet. Combining protein with carbohydrate stimulates muscle building to an even greater extent. Growth hormone is also stimulated by AstroBlast, which increases the rate of protein production, fat burning, and muscle growth.

Exercise and Hunger

After a good workout, you may feel hungry—and then become fearful that the calories you burned while exercising will quickly be replaced by those in the food you consume.

This is not the case. Research shows that most exercisers eat approximately the same amount of food as—or slightly more than—they would if they hadn't exercised. There is no evidence that exercise increases (or diminishes) appetite to any degree. To dispel guilt pangs: Remember that in many cases, the calories expended during an exercise session will exceed any appetite increase you might experience.

Snacks

Most meals satisfy your hunger for about two to three hours before hunger returns once again. As your blood sugar levels begin to dip, you may notice a slight decrease in your energy levels. To achieve the best results from the AstroFit program, your goal is not to feel hungry at any time throughout the day. Healthful snacking at the first signs of hunger pangs will help you achieve this aim.

Snacking on nutrient-rich foods such as fruits, vegetables, yogurt, and ready-to-eat cereals allows you to easily bridge the gaps between breakfast, lunch, and dinner, keeping your energy levels high throughout the day.

Think of your snacks as simple, easy-to-prepare minimeals that help replenish your blood sugar and muscle glycogen. Nutritious snacking takes some thought, so when you're making your weekly shopping list, be sure to include some of the items listed below. Keep these tasty items handy, whether in your cupboard, refrigerator, briefcase, glove compartment, office refrigerator, or purse.

The following are all high-carbohydrate, low-fat snacks that may be consumed *ad libitum*. Each contains less than 20 grams of fat (the snacks with an asterisk have no fat).

High-Carbohydrate Snacks

*Cereal and fruit bars
Chex Mix, reduced-fat
*Fruit
*Fruit, dried
*Fruit, frozen
*Fruit juice, unsweetened
Graham crackers
Granola bars, low-fat
Oatmeal Squares cereal
*Popcorn, *caramel, plain, or light natural microwave
*Popsicles
*Saltine crackers

*Sherbet
*Sorbet
*Vegetables, raw, with fat-free salad dressing
Tortilla chips, baked, with salsa
Yogurt, frozen, low-fat

Higher-Protein, High-Carbohydrate Snacks

Cottage cheese, 2 percent fat or lower, with fruit
Milk, chocolate, 1 percent fat or lower
Milk, skim
Saltines, with low-fat summer sausage
Yogurt, low-fat

Workout and Meal Schedules

People who exercise shortly after waking should eat differently from people who exercise just before bedtime. What time you eat your meals and snacks will vary according to when you want to exercise. Use this handy planner to help set your workout and eating timetable so you'll be able to perform at your best.

EARLY-MORNING WORKOUT/MEAL SCHEDULE

5:30 A.M.	PREWORKOUT SNACK
6:00 A.M.	WORKOUT, 6:00–6:30
7:00 A.M.	POSTWORKOUT SNACK OR BREAKFAST
9:30 A.M.	SNACK
NOON	LUNCH
3:00 P.M.	SNACK
6:00 P.M.	DINNER
9:00 P.M.	SNACK

MIDMORNING WORKOUT/MEAL SCHEDULE

7:00 A.M.	BREAKFAST
9:00 A.M.	PREWORKOUT SNACK
10:00 A.M.	WORKOUT, 10:30–11:00
11:30 A.M.	POSTWORKOUT SNACK OR LUNCH
3:00 P.M.	SNACK

| 6:00 P.M. | DINNER |
| 9:00 P.M. | SNACK |

NOON WORKOUT/MEAL SCHEDULE

7:00 A.M.	BREAKFAST
9:00 A.M.	SNACK
11:30 A.M.	PREWORKOUT SNACK
NOON	WORKOUT, NOON–12:30
1:00 P.M.	POSTWORKOUT SNACK OR LUNCH
3:00 P.M.	SNACK
6:00 P.M.	DINNER
9:00 P.M.	SNACK

MIDAFTERNOON WORKOUT/MEAL SCHEDULE

7:00 A.M.	BREAKFAST
9:30 A.M.	SNACK
NOON	LUNCH
2:30 P.M.	PREWORKOUT SNACK
3:00 P.M.	WORKOUT, 3:00–3:30
4:00 P.M.	POSTWORKOUT SNACK
6:00 P.M.	DINNER
9:00 P.M.	SNACK

LATE-AFTERNOON WORKOUT/MEAL SCHEDULE

7:00 A.M.	BREAKFAST
9:30 A.M.	SNACK
NOON	LUNCH
3:00 P.M.	SNACK
5:30 P.M.	PREWORKOUT SNACK
6:00 P.M.	WORKOUT, 6:00–6:30
7:00 P.M.	POSTWORKOUT SNACK
8:00 P.M.	DINNER
9:00 P.M.	SNACK

LATE-EVENING WORKOUT/MEAL SCHEDULE

7:00 A.M.	BREAKFAST
9:00 A.M.	SNACK
NOON	LUNCH
3:00 P.M.	SNACK
6:00 P.M.	DINNER
7:30 P.M.	PREWORKOUT SNACK
8:30 P.M.	WORKOUT, 8:30–9:00
9:15 P.M.	POSTWORKOUT SNACK

Don't Forget to Drink Water

Good nutrition includes drinking water throughout the day. Perspiration lost during a workout can cause poor performance. Lack of fluids or improper rehydration can lead to muscle cramping, early muscle fatigue, and, in extreme cases, nausea.

Blood—which is composed mainly of water—helps keep the major organs, the brain, and the skin at a steady temperature. The body has approximately 2.5 million sweat glands, and when they function properly, they excrete enough perspiration to keep you cool while exercising. However, if you don't replace this lost perspiration with water, your blood volume can drop, your body temperature can rise, and you will stop sweating altogether, leaving your body defenseless and susceptible to dehydration.

I strongly recommend that you drink a minimum of six eight-ounce glasses of fluid each day. When exercising, you should drink more, taking fluids every fifteen minutes during your workout, even if you don't feel thirsty. Cold water is absorbed faster than room-temperature water and will get to your bloodstream more quickly. Another plus: cold drinks absorb body heat internally and will cool you more quickly than room-temperature liquids.

Where to Get Help with Nutrition

You are bound to have additional dietary concerns regarding eating properly, how to lose body fat or put on muscle, or where specific nutritional changes can be made in your diet to enhance performance in a specific sport. In many instances, a sports nutritionist is a better source of information than your family physician. Most physicians have had little, if any, training in nutrition. Sports nutritionists are registered dietitians who have expertise in nutrition as it applies to exercise and can make dietary suggestions that will affect your health and performance in a positive way.

To make sure you receive advice from a qualified nutrition expert, consult a registered dietitian (R.D.) who is a member of the American Dietetic Association. For referrals to sports nutritionists in your area, call (800) 366-1655 from 9:00 A.M. to 4:00 P.M. (Central Time) Monday through Friday. This is a hotline operated by the National Center for Nutrition and Dietetics, a division of the American Dietetic Association.

Prepare Your AstroFit Shopping List

Planning varied and nutritious meals is critical. A well-stocked refrigerator and pantry will be a big help, so use this shopping list as a helpful reminder.

Fresh Produce

Apples	Grapes
Apricots	Nectarines
Avocados	Oranges
Bananas	Peaches
Berries	Pears
Cantaloupe	Plums
Grapefruit	

Vegetables

Asparagus	Eggplant
Artichokes	Garlic
Bell peppers	Green beans
Broccoli	Lettuce
Brussels sprouts	Mushrooms
Cabbage	Onions
Carrots	Potatoes
Cauliflower	Spinach
Celery	Sweet potatoes
Corn	Tomatoes
Cucumbers	Zucchini

Condiments

Mayonnaise, nonfat	Salsa
Mustard	Soy sauce
Salad dressing, nonfat	

Dairy Products (Low-Fat or Nonfat Only)

Cheese	Ice milk
Cottage cheese	Milk
Cream, sour	Tofu
Cream cheese	Yogurt
Egg substitute	Yogurt, frozen
Eggs (use whites for nonfat protein)	

Breads

Bagels	Rolls
Bread, whole wheat	Tortillas
English muffins	

Cereals

Granola	Shredded wheat
Oatmeal	Wheaties
Raisin or nut bran	

Staples

Almonds	Peanut butter
Beans, dry	Protein powder: whey or soy
Flour	Rice, brown
Fruit, dry	Rice, white
Lentils	Vegetable cooking spray
Olive oil	Wheat germ

Canned Products

Applesauce

Beans, black

Beans, garbanzo

Beans, kidney

Broth: chicken or beef

Peaches

Pears

Pineapple

Salmon

Sardines

Soup

Tomatoes

Tuna

Pasta

Macaroni

Noodles

Spaghetti

Meat/Poultry/Fish

Chicken, breast

Deli meats, lean

Fish fillets, fresh

Ground beef, lean

Ground turkey, lean

Ham, lean

Lamb, leg

Pork, tenderloin

Round steak

Sirloin steak

Scallops

Turkey, breast

Frozen Foods

Blueberries

Raspberries

Fruit juice bars

Microwave dinners, frozen

Juice, orange

Waffles

Peaches

Strawberries

Beverages

Coffee

Fruit juices, 100 percent

Tea

Tomato juice

Water, bottled

Snacks

Chips, low-fat

Crackers, whole wheat

Popcorn

Pretzels, whole wheat

Rice cakes

14

Eating for Optimal Health and Strength

The only real stumbling block is fear of failure.
In cooking you've got to have a what-the-hell attitude.
—JULIA CHILD

Welcome to the wonderful world of protein-rich eating that will help you build muscle, lose body fat, and keep you energized and happy.

Food is much more than something that placates that gnawing feeling in the pit of your stomach. Proper nutrition plays a critical role in how you look and feel. To achieve enduring success and health with AstroFit, you need to fuel your body with the right nutrients on a regular basis.

When it came to designing the AstroFit nutrition plan, I turned to Amanda Wells. Amanda is a registered dietitian, and for the past several years she has worked in my Nutrition, Metabolism, and Exercise Laboratory at the University of Arkansas for Medical Sciences. Amanda is currently the director of the Metabolic Kitchen, where she designs and implements metabolic research diets for all of our clinical research studies.

I discussed my 60-20-20 plan with her and gave her four guidelines I wanted her to keep in mind when she developed her meal plans:

- The meals should help to build lean body tissue and lose body fat.
- The recipes should be flavorful, high-energy, and easy to prepare.
- Meals should be designed with the novice chef in mind, but be exciting and tasty enough that people would look forward to them day after day.
- Each menu should contain complete nutrition information so that keeping track of the 60-20-20 breakdown and other important nutrition information is easy.

Amanda was intrigued by the challenge and developed fourteen daily menus, each containing about 2,500 calories of high-quality

Serving Sizes

Food	Serving Size
Breads, cereals, grains	1 slice bread
	1 pita pocket
	½ bagel
	½ bun
	½ English muffin
	1 bowl cereal
	2 large crackers
Vegetables	½ cup cooked or raw vegetables
	½ cup cooked legumes
Fruits	½ grapefruit
	1 medium piece of fruit
	¾ cup fruit juice
Milk	1 cup skim milk
	1.5 ounces cheese
	½ cup cottage cheese
Meat, poultry, fish	3 ounces cooked lean meat, poultry, or fish
	(the size of a deck of playing cards)

protein and complex carbohydrates. These low-fat daily menus are divided into three healthful meals. Each day's offerings provide exactly what's necessary from each of the food groups. With the energy from these nutritious meals, you will certainly meet all of your AstroFit goals.

You do not have to use Amanda's recipes in order to succeed with the AstroFit program. I have included them simply to prove to you that eating sensibly doesn't mean eliminating tasty, interesting foods from your diet.

Be aware that these food suggestions are not a magic formula for weight loss in and of themselves but are guidelines, basic suggestions about how you can work the 60-20-20 nutritional component of AstroFit so you can enjoy protein-rich, nutritious meals to complement your E-Centric workouts.

Feel free to adjust these recipes according to your own taste preferences and individual dietary concerns. Be creative, and above all, enjoy each meal. *Buon appetito!*

The AstroFit Meal Plan

Following are complete menus for fourteen days of AstroFit nutrition.

Day 1: Sunday

BREAKFAST
3 ounces plain bagel
3 ounces lox
1 cup skim milk
8 ounces orange juice

LUNCH
3 ounces grilled chicken breast
1 ounce slice of mozzarella cheese
1 hamburger bun
Lettuce
Tomato
1 teaspoon mustard
2 teaspoons mayonnaise
Baked Beans (p. 269)
1 ounce pretzels
12 ounces lemonade
1 Large apple

DINNER
2 Beef Fajitas (p. 259)
1 cup whole-kernel corn with red peppers
Jicama Slaw (p. 277)
Black Bean Salsa (p. 270)
1 ounce baked tortilla chips
1 cup skim milk
3 graham crackers

NUTRITION INFORMATION:

2,531 calories, 134 g Protein (21%), 382 g carbohydrate (60%), 56 g fat (20%), 1,362 mg calcium, 254 mg vitamin C, 3525 IU vitamin A, 12.5 IU vitamin E, 188 μg beta-carotene, 8 μg vitamin B12

Day 2: Monday

BREAKFAST
2 cups Strawberry Yogurt Smoothie (p. 278)
2 Oatmeal Muffins (p. 282)
1 tablespoon honey

LUNCH
Vegetable Beef Soup (p. 266)
1 Cornbread Muffin
Fruit Salad with Lime Poppy-Seed Dressing (p. 279)
1 cup skim milk

DINNER
6 ounces salmon
Garlic Mashed Potatoes (p. 274)
1 cup boiled or steamed asparagus
2 Whole-Wheat Rolls (p. 284)
2 tablespoons honey
1 slice angel food cake (1 ounce)
Peach Sauce (p. 281)
1 cup apple juice

NUTRITION INFORMATION

2,472 calories, 122 g protein (20%), 377 g carbohydrate (61%), 59 g fat (21%), 1,281 mg calcium, 169 mg vitamin C, 7,155 IU vitamin A, 8.9 IU vitamin E, 947 μg beta-carotene, 9.8 μg vitamin B12

Day 3: Tuesday

BREAKFAST
1 Omelet (p. 268)
2 slices whole-wheat toast
2 tablespoons jam or preserves
½ grapefruit with 1 tsp sugar
1 cup skim milk

LUNCH
2 slices rye bread
3 ounces turkey breast
Lettuce
Tomato
Pasta Salad (p. 272)
8 ounces vegetable or V8 juice
8 vanilla wafers
1 cup skim milk with 1 tablespoon chocolate syrup

DINNER
5 ounces pork tenderloin
1 cup Rice and Pasta (p. 272)
Glazed Carrots with Raisins (p. 275)
1 cup spinach with 2 teaspoons chopped green onions
1 tablespoon Russian dressing
1 cup orange sherbet
1 cup grapes

NUTRITION INFORMATION:
2,486 calories, 126 g protein (20%), 374 g carbohydrate (60%), 59 g fat (21%), 1,052 mg calcium, 202 mg vitamin C, 13,690 IU vitamin A, 14.0 IU vitamin E, 2,203 µg beta-carotene, 5.4 µg vitamin B12

Day 4: Wednesday

BREAKFAST

1 cup bran flakes with 1 cup skim milk
1 English muffin
1 tablespoon jam
1 banana
1 cup skim milk
1 cup orange juice

LUNCH

3 ounces sliced pork (leftover)
2 tablespoons barbecue sauce
1 hamburger bun
1 cup coleslaw
1 corn-on-the-cob niblets—1 small ear (~5 ounces)
1 cup cucumber with 1 tablespoon Italian dressing
1 cup watermelon

DINNER

4 ounces sirloin steak
1 baked potato
1 cup broccoli spears
2 Whole-Wheat Rolls (p. 284)
1 tablespoon butter
⅔ cup vanilla pudding
2 S'Mores (p. 285)

NUTRITION INFORMATION:

2,498 calories, 121 g protein (19%), 379 g carbohydrate (61%), 59 g fat (21%), 1,032 mg calcium, 191 mg vitamin C, 5,020 IU vitamin A, 11.0 IU vitamin E, 195 µg beta-carotene, 7.6 µg vitamin B12

Day 5: Thursday

BREAKFAST
2 slices French Toast (p. 283)
2 tablespoons powdered sugar
1 cup skim milk
1 cup apple juice

LUNCH
Steak Salad (p. 260)
10 saltine crackers
1 cup frozen presweetened strawberries, thawed

DINNER
Ginger Chicken (p. 262)
Fried Rice (p. 271)
1 cup steamed snow peas
Candied Sweet Potatoes (p. 275)
2 Betty's Cookies (p. 286)
1 pita bread
1 tablespoon honey
1 cup skim milk

NUTRITION INFORMATION:
2,494 calories, 134 g protein (21%), 373 g carbohydrate (60%), 57 g fat (21%), 1,142 mg calcium, 216 mg vitamin C, 10,625 IU vitamin A, 9.4 IU vitamin E, 1,799 µg beta-carotene, 6.1 µg vitamin B12

Day 6: Friday

BREAKFAST
1 English muffin
3 slices Canadian bacon
1 scrambled egg
1 orange
1 cup skim milk

LUNCH

4 ounces deli roast beef
2 slices whole-wheat bread
8 baby carrots
Marinated Potato Salad (p. 274)
1 cup pineapple, fresh or canned in juice

DINNER

Red Beans and Rice (p. 265)
1 Corn Muffin (p. 285)
Seasoned Yellow Squash (p. 278)
TofuBerry Smoothie (p. 278)

NUTRITION INFORMATION:

2,491 calories, 128 g protein (21%), 373 g carbohydrate (60%), 59 g fat (21%), 1,414 mg calcium, 288 mg vitamin C, 9,580 IU vitamin A, 14.2 IU vitamin E, 52 μg beta-carotene, 3.4 μg vitamin B12

Day 7: Saturday

BREAKFAST

1 cup oatmeal
1 cup raisins
1 slice whole-wheat bread
1 tablespoon butter
1 cup skim milk
1 cup orange juice

LUNCH

2 Chicken and Spinach Quesadillas (p. 262)
1 ounce baked tortilla chips
1 cup salsa
1 cup low-fat fruit yogurt
1 cereal and fruit bar

DINNER
3 Salmon Patties (p. 260)
1 cup green peas
Mashed Potatoes (p. 274)
2 Whole-Wheat Rolls (p. 284)
1 cup sliced plums
1 frozen fruit and juice bar

NUTRITION INFORMATION:
2,523 calories, 125 g protein (20%), 378 g carbohydrate (60%), 61 g fat (21%), 1,574 mg calcium, 208 mg vitamin C, 7,055 IU vitamin A, 13.41 IU vitamin E, 100 µg beta-carotene, 9.5 µg vitamin B12

Day 8: Sunday

BREAKFAST
3 Whole-Wheat Pancakes (p. 283)
1 cup Blueberry Syrup (p. 280)
3 slices Canadian bacon
1 cup skim milk

LUNCH
Macaroni and Bean Soup (p. 266)
10 saltine crackers
2 slices whole-wheat bread
2 tablespoons reduced-fat peanut butter mixed with
    1 tablespoon corn syrup
1 apple

DINNER
1 6-ounce lamb chop
Stewed Okra and Tomatoes (p. 277)
1 cup black-eyed peas
1 slice whole-wheat bread
1 slice angel food cake with 2 ounces canned cherry pie filling

1 tablespoon nondairy whipped topping
Apricot Salad (p. 280)
1 cup skim milk

NUTRITION INFORMATION:
2,518 calories, 134 g protein (21%), 382 g carbohydrate (61%), 58 g fat (21%), 1,421 mg calcium, 76 mg vitamin C, 8,515 IU vitamin A, 12.1 IU vitamin E, 869 µg beta-carotene, 7.8 µg vitamin B12

Day 9: Monday

BREAKFAST
1 cup Fiber One cereal
1 cup blueberries
1 cup skim milk
2 slices whole-wheat toast
1 tablespoon butter
1 cup cranberry juice

LUNCH
5 ounces tunafish
1 tablespoon mayonnaise
1 tablespoon pickle relish
2 slices whole-wheat bread
1 ounce pretzels
1 cup canned fruit cocktail in light syrup

DINNER
Chicken Spaghetti (p. 263)
1 cup green beans
2 Crumb Topped Tomato Halves (p. 277)
2 bread sticks
Banana Pudding (p. 281)
2 slices pumpernickel bread
2 ounces (¼ cup) Tofu Spinach Dip (p. 276)
1 cup skim milk

NUTRITION INFORMATION:
2,498 calories, 131 g protein (21%), 380 g carbohydrate (61%), 59 g fat (21%), 1,262 mg calcium, 127 mg vitamin C, 4,790 IU vitamin A, 16.9 IU vitamin E, 346 µg beta-carotene, 6.6 µg vitamin B12

Day 10: Tuesday

BREAKFAST
1 cinnamon raisin bagel
1 ounce Neufchâtel cheese
½ grapefruit with 1 teaspoon sugar
1 cup skim milk

LUNCH
Corn Chowder (p. 267)
4 ounces sliced ham
2 slices rye bread
1 teaspoon mustard
Lettuce
Tomato
1 cup skim milk
4 fig bar cookies

DINNER
Baked Halibut (p. 264)
Broccoli and Pasta (p. 272)
2 Whole-Wheat Rolls (p. 284)
1 tablespoon butter
Fruit Trifle (p. 280)
2 cups plain popcorn
1 cup grape juice

NUTRITION INFORMATION:
2,495 calories, 125 g protein (20%), 380 g carbohydrate (61%), 57 g fat (20%), 1,294 mg calcium, 241 mg vitamin C, 4,620 IU vitamin A, 9.8 IU vitamin E, 259 µg beta-carotene, 4.6 µg vitamin B12

Day 11: Wednesday

BREAKFAST
Breakfast Bake (p. 269)
1 cup skim milk
1 cup orange juice

LUNCH
4 ounces baked chicken breast
1 cup cooked pasta
1 cup Chunky Garden Style Spaghetti Sauce
1 cup creamed corn
2 bread sticks
1 cup sliced fresh pears

DINNER
5 ounces baked ham
Spinach Salad with Mandarin Oranges (p. 276)
Candied Sweet Potatoes (p. 275)
Confetti Wild Rice Pilaf (p. 271)
1 slice whole-wheat bread
2 cups Soy Milk Piña Colada Smoothie (p. 279)

NUTRITION INFORMATION:
2,499 calories, 128 g protein (20%), 383 g carbohydrate (61%), 56 g fat (20%), 809 mg calcium, 266 mg vitamin C, 16,270 IU vitamin A, 11.5 IU vitamin E, 2,548 μg beta-carotene, 3.2 μg vitamin B12

Day 12: Thursday

BREAKFAST
1 cup Cream of Wheat
1 cup skim milk
1 cup raisins
2 slices whole-wheat bread
1 tablespoon jam
1 cup apple juice

LUNCH

Chili (p. 267)
1 cup oyster crackers
1 cup melon
3 tablespoons Yogurt Fruit Topping (p. 281)
1 cup skim milk

DINNER

6 ounces Roast Beef (p. 265)
1 cup Roasted Potatoes
1 cup Roasted Carrots and Onions
1 cup brussels sprouts
2 dinner rolls
1 fruit and cereal bar
1 cup dried fruit

NUTRITION INFORMATION:

2,484 calories, 127 g protein (20%), 375 g carbohydrate (60%), 58 g fat (21%), 1,144 mg calcium, 144 mg vitamin C, 15,005 IU vitamin A, 11.0 IU vitamin E, 2,253 µg beta-carotene, 7.7 µg vitamin B12

Day 13: Friday

BREAKFAST

2 Fiber One muffins
1 scrambled egg
1 cup honeydew melon
1 cup skim milk
1 cup orange juice

LUNCH

3 ounces broiled hamburger patty
1 hamburger bun
Baked Beans (p. 269)
Baked Fries (p. 273)
1 cup tropical fruit salad canned in juice

DINNER
Lemon Pepper Chicken (p. 264)
1 cup broccoli
Couscous and Tomatoes (p. 273)
1 slice whole-wheat bread
1 cup skim milk
4 Betty's Cookies (p. 286)
10 slices red and green bell peppers
1 celery stalk
4 baby carrots
2 tablespoons ranch dressing

NUTRITION INFORMATION:
2,529 calories, 136 g protein (21%), 383 g carbohydrate (61%), 58 g fat (21%), 1,261 mg calcium, 469 mg vitamin C, 8,285 IU vitamin A, 17.9 IU vitamin E, 160 µg beta-carotene, 5.8 µg vitamin B12

Day 14: Saturday

BREAKFAST
1 cup Cheerios
1 banana
1 cup skim milk
8 ounces low-fat yogurt
1 English muffin
2 teaspoons butter

LUNCH
2 slices rye bread
3 ounces turkey
1 cup sprouts
2 slices tomato
Hummus (p. 270)
1 pita bread, split and toasted
1 orange
1 cup skim milk

DINNER

Herbed Shrimp and Fettuccine (p. 261)
1 cup asparagus
1 cup acorn squash
1 tablespoon butter
1 slice French bread
1 slice "Cheese" Cake (p. 286)
2 tablespoons canned pie filling
1 cup fat-free cottage cheese
1 cup sliced fresh peaches

NUTRITION INFORMATION:

2,483 calories, 130 g protein (21%), 383 g carbohydrate (61%), 55 g fat (20%), 1,338 mg calcium, 255 mg vitamin C, 4,475 IU vitamin A, 9.4 IU vitamin E, 196 µg beta-carotene, 5.0 µg vitamin B12

AstroFit Recipes

BEEF FAJITAS

Makes 8 fajitas

1 pound sirloin or flank steak

1 cup salsa

1 tablespoon canola oil

2 tablespoons lemon or lime juice

1 teaspoon Worcestershire sauce

1 teaspoon chili powder

8 eight-inch flour tortillas

1 large sliced onion

1 sliced green bell pepper

1 chopped ripe tomato

Place beef in the freezer and allow it to partially freeze (30 minutes to 1 hour). Remove from freezer and slice thinly across the grain into strips. Place strips into a plastic zipper bag. Pour the salsa, oil, lemon juice, Worcestershire sauce, and chili powder over the beef. Seal the bag and shake to coat the beef with seasonings. Place the bag in a shallow dish in the refrigerator and allow the beef to marinate for 1 to 24 hours.

Once the meat has marinated, wrap the tortillas in foil and heat in a 350-degree oven for 10 minutes. While the tortillas are warming, preheat a large nonstick skillet. Place the undrained meat into the hot skillet. Cook and stir for 2 to 3 minutes, then add the onion. Cook for another 3 minutes, then add the sliced bell pepper. Cook for an additional 2 to 3 minutes. Stir in the chopped tomato.

To serve, fill the warm tortillas with the beef mixture. Top with additional salsa if desired.

SALMON PATTIES

Makes 10 patties

2 eggs

15 ounces canned salmon, drained

1 cup finely chopped onion

1 cup bread crumbs

1 tablespoon prepared mustard

In a small bowl, beat the eggs lightly with a fork. Add all other ingredients and stir until well mixed. Preheat a nonstick skillet. Use a ⅓ cup measuring cup to scoop the mixture. Place the scoops of mixture in the skillet, flattening with the back of the measuring cup. Cook for 4 minutes on low heat until golden brown. Turn over and cook on other side for another 4 minutes.

STEAK SALAD

Makes 2 salads

⅓ cup olive oil

4 ounces red wine vinegar

2 tablespoons lemon juice

1 teaspoon garlic salt

1 teaspoon dried thyme

1 teaspoon dried marjoram

1 teaspoon black pepper

8 ounces steak, cooked (use leftovers if available)

2 cups lettuce

1 grated carrot

1 cup sliced mushrooms

6 cherry tomatoes, halved

In a plastic zipper bag, combine the oil, vinegar, lemon juice, and herbs and spices. Add the cooked steak. Close the bag and shake to coat. Let sit for 15 to 30 minutes. Meanwhile, divide the lettuce into two portions and top with the carrots, mushrooms, and halved tomatoes. Place the steak on top of the prepared vegetables. Serve cold.

HERBED SHRIMP AND FETTUCCINE

Makes 4 servings

6 ounces uncooked fettuccine

2 cups sliced mushrooms

1 cup chopped onions

2 minced garlic cloves

1 tablespoon olive oil

1 cup chicken broth

1 teaspoon cornstarch

1 teaspoon dried basil

1 teaspoon dried oregano

¼ teaspoon black pepper

12 ounces shrimp, peeled and deveined

2 diced tomatoes

1 cup grated Parmesan cheese

Cook the fettuccine according to the package directions. Drain and keep warm. In a large saucepan sauté the mushrooms, onions, and garlic in oil until the onion is tender. In a small mixing bowl, combine the broth, cornstarch, and herbs and spices. Add to the mushroom mixture. Cook and stir until thickened and bubbly. Add the shrimp and simmer covered, about 2 minutes. Stir in the tomatoes and heat through. Spoon the mixture over the pasta and sprinkle with Parmesan cheese. Toss to coat.

GINGER CHICKEN

Makes 4 servings

4 chicken breasts

2 tablespoons soy sauce

2 tablespoons vinegar

1 teaspoon dried ginger

1 teaspoon garlic powder

1 cup water

Place all the ingredients in a plastic zipper bag. Shake to coat. Marinate for 30 minutes to 1 hour. Bake the chicken at 350 degrees for 30 minutes or until done.

CHICKEN AND SPINACH QUESADILLAS

Makes 4 servings

1 cup diced tomatoes with green chilies

2 cups cooked diced chicken

1 cup shredded cheddar cheese

10 ounces frozen chopped spinach, thawed

8 flour tortillas

Squeeze the spinach to remove excess liquid. Combine the tomatoes, chicken, and cheese with the spinach. Divide the mixture among the tortillas. Fold the topped tortillas. Cook over low heat on a non-stick griddle or skillet, turning occasionally, until heated through.

CHICKEN SPAGHETTI

Makes 8 servings

4 ounces uncooked spaghetti

1 teaspoon flour

1 cup skim milk

1 pound chicken, stewed and diced

1 cup 98% fat-free cream of mushroom soup

2 ounces sliced mushrooms

1 teaspoon salt

1 cup red bell pepper

Vegetable spray

Cook the spaghetti according to the package directions. Place the flour in a cup and slowly stir in the milk, making sure there are no lumps. In a large mixing bowl, combine the cooked chicken, cooked spaghetti, milk-and-flour mixture, and other ingredients. Spray a large baking dish with vegetable spray and spoon the mixture evenly into the dish. Bake at 350 degrees for 40 to 45 minutes or until heated through.

BAKED HALIBUT

Makes 8 servings

8 four-ounce halibut steaks

1 tablespoon Dijon mustard

1 cup lemon juice

1 tablespoon vinegar

1 teaspoon dried oregano

1 teaspoon black pepper

1 cup water or chicken broth

2 sliced green onions

Rinse and dry the halibut steaks. Place in a shallow baking dish. Brush with the mustard. Combine the lemon juice, vinegar, oregano, pepper, and water or broth. Pour over the fish. Marinate in refrigerator for 1 to 2 hours. Top the fish with the green onion. Bake at 375 degrees for 25 minutes or until fish flakes easily.

LEMON PEPPER CHICKEN

Makes 7 servings

1 pound skinless chicken breasts

1 tablespoon soy sauce

1 tablespoon lemon pepper seasoning

Combine all ingredients in a plastic zipper bag. Shake until the chicken is evenly coated. Place the chicken in a baking dish and bake at 350 degrees for 45 minutes or until done.

Roast Beef with Roasted Potatoes, Carrots, and Onions

Makes 8 servings

3 pounds beef chuck roast

Garlic powder

Salt

Black pepper

½ cup water

8 small potatoes, peeled and quartered

8 carrots, peeled and cut into 2-inch pieces

2 onions cut into wedges

Trim fat from roast. Sprinkle with garlic powder, salt, and black pepper to cover all sides of roast. In an electric skillet over high heat sear all sides of the roast until browned. Reduce heat and allow roast to simmer with added water, covered, for 1 hour 15 minutes. Turn roast over. Add potatoes, carrots, and onions and cook, covered, for an additional 45 minutes.

Red Beans and Rice

Makes 4 servings

1 cup dry kidney beans

1 pound low-fat smoked sausage

3 cups water

1 chopped onion

1 teaspoon bay leaf

3 tablespoons soy sauce

1 tablespoon chili powder

1 teaspoon black pepper

2 cups cooked rice

Sort and wash the beans. Combine all the ingredients except rice in a slow cooker and simmer 8 hours. Combine with the rice.

VEGETABLE BEEF SOUP

Makes 4 servings

1 pound ground beef

1 chopped small onion

4 cups whole tomatoes

1 stalk diced celery

1 peeled and diced potato

2 peeled and sliced carrots

2 cups canned green beans

2 ounces uncooked macaroni

Brown the beef and onion together. Drain off the fat. Add the tomatoes and other vegetables. Bring mixture to a boil. Cover. Reduce heat and simmer for 20 minutes, stirring occasionally. Stir in the macaroni and continue to cook for an additional 15 minutes or until the macaroni is done.

MACARONI AND BEAN SOUP

Makes 6 servings

2 sliced carrots

2 stalks diced celery

1 chopped medium onion

3 tablespoons olive oil

1 15-ounce can tomatoes

1 14½-ounce can chicken broth

1 teaspoon salt

1 teaspoon pepper

3 cups water

1 14½-ounce can white kidney beans

1 14½-ounce can red kidney beans

1 cup cooked macaroni

1 package (10 ounces) frozen spinach

In a Dutch oven or large saucepan, sauté the carrots, celery, and onion in the oil until tender. Add the tomatoes, broth, salt, pepper, and water. Heat to boiling. Reduce heat and simmer uncovered for 10 minutes. Drain the kidney beans and mash the white kidney beans. Add all the beans, the cooked macaroni, and the spinach. Cook over medium heat until heated through.

CHILI

Makes 4 servings

1 pound lean ground beef

1 cup chopped onions

1 cup chopped bell pepper

2 minced garlic cloves

16 ounces stewed tomatoes

1 16-ounce can red kidney beans

8 ounces tomato sauce

3 teaspoons chili powder

In a Dutch oven or large saucepan, brown the beef, onions, pepper, and garlic. Drain off the fat. Add the remaining ingredients. Heat to boiling. Reduce heat and simmer, covered, for 30 minutes, stirring occasionally.

CORN CHOWDER

Makes 4 servings

1 chopped onion

1 cup water

3 peeled and diced potatoes

1 16-ounce can sweet corn

2 cups skim milk

2 tablespoons all-purpose flour

1 teaspoon black pepper

In a large saucepan, combine the onion, water, potatoes, and corn. Bring to a boil. Reduce heat, cover, and simmer for 10 minutes, until potatoes are tender. Pour in 1 cup of the milk. In a small bowl, combine the remaining milk, the flour, and the pepper. Slowly add this to the corn mixture. Cook and stir until mixture is heated through and thickened.

OMELET

Makes 1

1 teaspoon canola oil

2 tablespoons chopped onion

1 tablespoon chopped bell pepper

1 whole large egg

2 egg whites

1 tablespoon water

Salt

Pepper

1 small diced ripe tomato

Coat a small nonstick skillet with the oil. Sauté the onion and bell pepper until tender. Remove from pan. In a bowl, beat together the egg, egg whites, and water. Pour into a hot pan. Cook the mixture over low heat, gently lifting the edges and tilting the pan. When egg is almost set, season to taste with salt and pepper, then spoon on the onion, bell pepper, and tomatoes. Loosen the edges, fold the omelet in half, and cook for 1 minute more. Slide the omelet out of the pan and onto a plate.

BREAKFAST BAKE

Makes 4 servings

Vegetable cooking spray

4 slices whole-wheat bread

1 cup frozen diced potatoes

4 slices Canadian bacon

1 cup shredded mozzarella

2 sliced green onions

1 cup diced bell pepper

3 beaten eggs

1 cup skim milk

1 teaspoon ground mustard

¼ teaspoon black pepper

Coat an 8" × 8" baking dish with vegetable cooking spray. Layer the bread, potatoes, bacon, cheese, onions, and peppers in the dish. Mix together the eggs, milk, mustard, and pepper. Pour over layers. Bake in at 325 degrees for about 25 minutes, until the eggs are firm.

BAKED BEANS

Makes 4 servings

2 15-ounce cans navy beans in tomato sauce

1 cup chopped onion

1 finely diced medium green bell pepper

1 tablespoon prepared mustard

2 tablespoons brown sugar

Combine the beans, onion, and pepper in a small glass dish. Stir in the mustard and brown sugar. Bake uncovered at 350 degrees for 40 minutes or microwave for 20 minutes (stirring after 10 minutes).

BLACK BEAN SALSA

Makes 4 servings

1 15-ounce can black beans, rinsed and drained

1 cup whole-kernel corn

1 small diced purple onion

1 diced ripe firm tomato, such as Roma

2 tablespoons chopped fresh cilantro

2 tablespoons lime juice

1 tablespoon olive oil

1 tablespoon vinegar

1 teaspoon salt

1 teaspoon black pepper

Combine all the ingredients. Mix well and serve.

Note: This can be made in advance and placed in the refrigerator to chill. Add the tomatoes just before serving to prevent them from becoming mushy. You also can omit the cilantro and serve as a side salad.

HUMMUS

Makes 5 servings

1 15-ounce can garbanzo beans

3 tablespoons peanut butter

3 tablespoons lemon juice

2 minced garlic cloves

1 teaspoon paprika

Drain the liquid from beans. Process until smooth in a blender or food processor. Add the other ingredients and mix until well combined. Chill.

FRIED RICE

Makes 4 servings

2 eggs, beaten

3 cups cooked rice, chilled

1 teaspoon ginger

2 cups shredded cabbage

1 cup green peas

1 cup sliced green onions

2 tablespoons soy sauce

Pour the eggs into a preheated nonstick skillet. When partially set, stir to break into pieces and add the other ingredients. Stir frequently and cook until the cabbage is tender.

CONFETTI WILD RICE PILAF

Makes 6 cups

1 4-ounce package (⅔ cup) wild rice

1 chicken flavor bouillon cube

3¾ cups water

1 bunch green onions, chopped

2 carrots, chopped

1 red bell pepper, chopped

3 tablespoons butter

¼ teaspoon salt

1 cup long-grain rice, uncooked

¼ cup chopped fresh parsley

In a large saucepan combine wild rice, bouillon cube, and water. Bring to a boil. Reduce heat to low, cover, and simmer for 25 minutes. While rice is simmering, sauté vegetables with butter and salt in a small skillet until lightly browned, about 10 minutes. Set aside. After wild rice has simmered 25 minutes, stir in long-grain rice. Heat to boiling, reduce heat to low, cover, and simmer for 20 minutes, or until all liquid is absorbed. Stir in parsley and cooked vegetables.

RICE AND PASTA

Makes 10 servings

2 cups uncooked long-grain rice

4 ounces uncooked orzo

1 finely chopped onion

32 ounces beef consommé

1 teaspoon black pepper

Combine all the ingredients in a large saucepan. Bring to a boil. Cover and reduce heat to low. Cook for 15 minutes. Remove pan from heat and allow to set for 5 minutes. Remove lid and stir.

PASTA SALAD

Makes 4 servings

1 cup Italian dressing

2 cups cooked and cooled multicolored rotini or small shell pasta

1 medium chopped tomato

1 tablespoon chopped black olives

Pour the Italian dressing over the pasta. Mix until evenly coated. Fold in the tomato and olives. Chill.

BROCCOLI AND PASTA

Makes 4 servings

1 tablespoon olive oil

1 teaspoon garlic powder

2 cups broccoli, cut into bite-size pieces

2 cups cooked bowtie pasta

2 tablespoons grated Parmesan cheese

In a large nonstick skillet, combine the broccoli, oil and garlic powder. Cook over medium heat until the broccoli is firm but tender. Stir in the pasta and cook until heated through. Remove from heat and top with Parmesan cheese.

COUSCOUS AND TOMATOES

Makes 4 servings

1 14-ounce can stewed tomatoes

1 cup water

1 cup chopped onions

⅛ teaspoon cayenne pepper

⅛ teaspoon garlic powder

1 cup uncooked couscous

In a saucepan, combine the tomatoes, water, onion, and spices. Bring to a boil. Stir in couscous. Cover and remove from heat. Let stand 5 minutes. Stir and serve.

BAKED FRIES

Makes 5 servings

5 baking potatoes

2 egg whites

Vegetable spray

Peel the potatoes and cut them into strips. In a large bowl, beat the egg whites slightly. Add the potatoes and mix, coating the potatoes. Spray a baking sheet with the vegetable spray and spread the potatoes in a thin layer. Bake potatoes in a 400-degree oven for 40 minutes, turning potatoes with a spatula every 6 to 8 minutes.

MARINATED POTATO SALAD

Makes 4 servings

1 pound small new potatoes

1 cup oil and vinegar salad dressing

1 diced bell pepper

6 halved cherry tomatoes

1 sliced red onion

Boil the potatoes. Cool and cut into quarters. Pour the dressing over the potatoes and mix in the other vegetables. Chill.

MASHED POTATOES

Makes 4 servings

1 pound potatoes

1 teaspoon salt

1 teaspoon dried parsley

Peel and quarter the potatoes. Place in a saucepan with the salt and just enough water to cover. Heat to boiling and boil for 20 minutes. Drain off some of the liquid, if desired. Mash potatoes with a potato masher or beat with a mixer. Sprinkle with parsley.

GARLIC MASHED POTATOES

Makes 4 servings

1 pound small potatoes

1 teaspoon salt

2 teaspoons butter

1 teaspoon garlic powder

1 teaspoon dried parsley

Peel and quarter the potatoes. In a saucepan, cover them with water, add the salt and boil for 20 to 25 minutes or until you are able to easily stick a fork through them. Drain off the liquid and set aside. Add the butter, garlic powder, and parsley to the potatoes and mash with a potato masher or beat with an electric mixer on low speed. Add reserved liquid as necessary to achieve the desired consistency.

GLAZED CARROTS WITH RAISINS

Makes 4 servings

6 large carrots
2 tablespoons brown sugar
2 tablespoons lemon juice
1 cup raisins

Peel and slice the carrots. Simmer in boiling water (just covering carrots) for about 15 minutes. Allow most of the water to evaporate, then add the brown sugar, lemon juice, and raisins. Continue to cook slowly over low heat until glazed.

CANDIED SWEET POTATOES

Makes 4 servings

3 sweet potatoes, peeled and sliced
2 tablespoons brown sugar
1 tablespoon butter

Combine all the ingredients and microwave for 20 minutes or until the potatoes are done, stirring every 5 minutes.

SPINACH SALAD WITH MANDARIN ORANGES

Makes 4 servings

1 tablespoon olive oil

1 tablespoon lemon juice

1 tablespoon honey

¼ teaspoon garlic powder

1 cup torn spinach leaves

1 cup mandarin oranges

In a small bowl, combine the oil, lemon juice, honey, and garlic powder. In a larger bowl combine the spinach and oranges. Pour the dressing over the spinach mixture and toss to coat.

TOFU SPINACH DIP

Makes 2 cups

12 ounces firm silken tofu

4 tablespoons plain nonfat yogurt

1 packet vegetable soup mix, dry

1 cup fat-free mayonnaise

10 ounces chopped frozen spinach, thawed

4 thinly sliced green onions

In a small bowl, mash the tofu. Stir in the yogurt, soup mix, and mayonnaise and mix well. Stir in the spinach and green onions. Chill.

JICAMA SLAW

Makes 4 servings

1 cup shredded cabbage

1 cup grated jicama

1 grated medium carrot

2 tablespoons mayonnaise

1 tablespoon lime juice or vinegar

1 teaspoon chili powder

Peel and grate the jicama and carrot. Add shredded cabbage. Mix in the mayonnaise and lime juice. Sprinkle with the chili powder. Serve chilled.

CRUMB-TOPPED TOMATO HALVES

Makes 2 servings

2 red tomatoes

2 tablespoons seasoned bread crumbs

Vegetable cooking spray

Wash and core the tomatoes, then cut them in half. Place the halves in a baking dish with the cut side up. Top with the bread crumbs, then spray lightly with vegetable cooking spray. Bake at 375 degrees for 15 minutes.

STEWED OKRA AND TOMATOES

Makes 4 servings

1 finely diced onion

1 pound sliced okra

3 large tomatoes

⅛ teaspoon black pepper

1 teaspoon salt

Combine all the ingredients in a large saucepan. Cook, covered, until the okra is tender.

SEASONED YELLOW SQUASH

Makes 4 servings

2 cups sliced yellow squash

1 cup diced onion

1 teaspoon black pepper

1 teaspoon salt

Combine the squash and onion in a microwave-safe dish. Microwave on high for 10 minutes. Stir in the pepper and salt. Microwave for an additional 5 minutes, or until the squash is tender.

STRAWBERRY YOGURT SMOOTHIE

Makes 4 servings

8 ounces nonfat vanilla yogurt

1 cup skim milk

1 cup strawberries, fresh or frozen

2 tablespoons powdered sugar

Combine all the ingredients in a blender and blend until smooth.

TOFUBERRY SMOOTHIE

Makes 2 servings

5 ounces firm silken tofu

2 tablespoons soy milk

1 cup vanilla nonfat yogurt

1 cup sweetened frozen raspberries

1 banana

2 cups orange juice

Combine all the ingredients in a blender and blend until smooth.

SOY MILK PIÑA COLADA SMOOTHIE

Makes 4 servings

2 bananas

1 cup pineapple

1 cup vanilla soy milk

3 dates

1 tablespoon coconut flakes

2 tablespoons maple syrup

Combine all the ingredients in a blender and blend until smooth.

FRUIT SALAD WITH LIME POPPY-SEED DRESSING

Makes 4 servings

1 cup seedless red grapes, halved

1 cup chopped Yellow Delicious apple

1 cup chopped green pear

1 cup pineapple chunks

1 cup limeade concentrate, thawed

1 cup honey

1 tablespoon poppy seeds

Combine all the fruit. Add the limeade concentrate, honey, and poppy seeds. Stir until the fruit is evenly coated. Can be chilled or served as is.

APRICOT SALAD

Makes 5 servings

1 cup boiling water

1 3-ounce package apricot or orange gelatin mix

5.5 ounces apricot nectar

2 tablespoons lemon juice

⅓ cup nonfat vanilla yogurt

4 apricots, peeled and chopped

In a mixing bowl, combine the boiling water and gelatin mix. Stir until the gelatin is dissolved. Stir in the apricot nectar and lemon juice. Chill until partially set. Beat with a mixer 1 to 2 minutes, until fluffy. Beat in the yogurt. Fold in the apricots and chill until firm.

FRUIT TRIFLE

Makes 4 servings

4 slices angel food cake

1 cup sweetened, sliced strawberries

1 sliced banana

1 cup vanilla pudding

1 cup canned cherry pie filling

Tear the cake into pieces and place in a small serving bowl. Layer fruit, then pudding. Spread the pie filling on top. Chill.

BLUEBERRY SYRUP

Makes 2 cups

1 cup blueberries

⅔ cup sugar

2 tablespoons cornstarch

⅛ teaspoon salt

2 tablespoons lemon juice

1 cup water

In a small saucepan, combine the blueberries, sugar, cornstarch, salt, and lemon juice. Mix until the berries are well coated. Slowly add the water, mixing well. Heat over medium heat, stirring frequently until thickened.

PEACH SAUCE

Makes 4 servings

1 tablespoon cornstarch

1 cup orange juice

1 10-ounce can peaches

1 teaspoon ground cinnamon

Combine the cornstarch and orange juice. Pour over the peaches. Microwave for 5 minutes. Stir in the cinnamon.

YOGURT FRUIT TOPPING

Makes 1½ cups

8 ounce nonfat vanilla yogurt

½ cup nondairy whipped topping

Placed yogurt in a small bowl. Fold in whipped topping. Chill.

BANANA PUDDING

Makes 4 servings

2 sliced bananas

1 3-ounce package instant vanilla pudding prepared with skim milk

16 vanilla wafers

Combine the bananas and pudding. Place four vanilla wafers in each of four dessert dishes. Top with the pudding mixture.

OATMEAL MUFFINS

Makes 12 muffins

1 cup quick oats

1 cup buttermilk

1 large egg, beaten

2 tablespoons canola oil

1 cup brown sugar

1 cup self-rising flour

¼ teaspoon baking soda

Preheat oven to 350 degrees. Place the oats in a mixing bowl. Pour the buttermilk over the oats and let stand for 5 to 10 minutes. Stir in the egg and oil until mixed. Stir in the sugar and the flour mixed with the baking soda. Mix lightly. Drop by spoonfuls into paper-lined muffin tins.

FIBER ONE MUFFINS

Makes 12 muffins

1 cup Fiber One cereal

1 cup skim milk

1 large egg, beaten

2 tablespoons canola oil

1 tablespoon honey

1 cup all-purpose flour

2 teaspoons baking powder

1 teaspoon salt

1 teaspoon ground cinnamon

In a small mixing bowl, combine the cereal and milk. Let stand for 10 minutes. Stir in the egg, oil, and honey. Sift together the dry ingredients. Stir into the cereal mixture until lumpy. Pour the batter into prepared muffin cups. Bake at 350 degrees for 20 to 25 minutes.

WHOLE-WHEAT PANCAKES

Makes 8 pancakes

1 cup whole-wheat flour

1 tablespoon sugar

2 teaspoons baking powder

1 teaspoon salt

1 egg, beaten

1 cup skim milk

1 tablespoon canola oil

In a small bowl, sift the dry ingredients together. Stir in the egg, milk, and oil until well blended. Ladle batter onto a preheated nonstick skillet or griddle. Cook over low heat until the top begins to set around the edges. Flip and cook on other side until done.

FRENCH TOAST

Makes 8 slices

1 large egg

2 egg whites

1 cup skim milk

¼ teaspoon ground cinnamon

8 slices French bread

Beat the eggs with milk and cinnamon. Dip the bread in the egg mixture, coating both sides. Place in a preheated nonstick skillet. Cook over low heat until golden brown on both sides.

WHOLE-WHEAT ROLLS

Makes 24 rolls

1 cup 2% fat, creamed cottage cheese

1 cup skim milk

1 package dry active yeast

4 cups whole-wheat flour

⅓ cup brown sugar

1 cup canola oil

2 large eggs, beaten

Drain the cottage cheese and reserve the liquid. Add the milk to the liquid to equal 1 cup. Combine the yeast and salt with 1 cup of the flour. Stir together the cottage cheese, liquid, sugar, oil, and beaten eggs and heat until warm.

Beat in flour and yeast mixture with an electric mixer on low speed for 30 seconds. Beat on high for 3 minutes, scraping sides of bowl.

With spoon, stir in as much remaining flour as possible. Turn dough onto floured surface. Knead in enough remaining flour to make a moderately stiff dough that is smooth and elastic. Shape into a ball. Place dough in a greased bowl and turn once, so surface of dough is not dry. Cover and let rise in a warm place about 40 minutes, until double in size. Punch dough down. Turn onto a lightly floured surface. Cover and let rest for 10 minutes. Shape into 24 smooth balls. Place balls in a greased 9" × 13" pan. Let rise in a warm place till almost double, about 20 minutes. Bake at 375 degrees for 15 minutes.

CORN MUFFINS

Makes 12 muffins

1 cup yellow or white cornmeal

1 cup all-purpose flour

2 tablespoons sugar

1 tablespoon baking powder

1 teaspoon salt

2 large eggs, beaten

1 cup skim milk

2 tablespoons canola oil

Preheat oven to 425 degrees. Sift together the cornmeal, flour, sugar, baking powder, and salt into a small mixing bowl. Stir in the eggs, milk, and oil until well mixed. Spray the bottoms of a twelve-muffin tin, or line the tin with paper muffin cups. Divide batter into twelve muffins. Bake for 20 to 25 minutes until golden brown.

S'MORES

Makes 6 servings

12 graham crackers

1 chocolate bar

6 large marshmallows

Place the graham crackers on a cookie sheet. Divide the chocolate bar into twelve pieces. Top each of six crackers with one piece of chocolate and one marshmallow. Top the other six crackers with a piece of chocolate. Broil for a few minutes, until marshmallow is toasted and chocolate begins to melt. Place each of the halves together, combining one with a marshmallow and one without a marshmallow.

BETTY'S COOKIES

Makes 2 dozen cookies

3 egg whites
1 teaspoon salt
1 cup powdered sugar
1 tablespoon all-purpose flour
1 cup chopped dates
1 teaspoon vanilla

Beat the egg whites and salt until stiff. Mix the powdered sugar and flour together. Add to the stiffened egg whites a spoonful at a time, continuing to beat until very stiff. Fold in the dates and vanilla. Drop by the teaspoon onto a cookie sheet lined with parchment paper or a paper bag. Bake for 30 minutes at 300 degrees. Let cool in pan 5 minutes before removing.

"CHEESE" CAKE

Makes 8 servings

1 cup pineapple juice
2 tablespoons unflavored gelatin
2 tablespoons butter
1 cup graham cracker crumbs
1 pound soft, silken tofu
5 tablespoons honey
6 tablespoons lemon juice

In a small saucepan, heat the pineapple juice until warm. Sprinkle the gelatin into warm juice. Stir until dissolved and let sit for 10 minutes.

Make the crust: Microwave the butter in a glass pie plate until mostly melted. Add the graham cracker crumbs. Mix until well combined, then spread the crumbs evenly in the bottom and up the sides of the pie plate. Microwave for 30 seconds.

In a blender, combine the tofu, honey, and lemon juice. Pour in the cooled pineapple juice–gelatin mixture. Blend until smooth. Pour the mixture into the crust. Refrigerate for 2 to 4 hours.

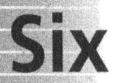

Six

Gauging Your Success

15

Looking Ahead

Only those who risk going too far can possibly find out how far one can go.
—T.S. Eliot

AstroFit is based on the most current research designed to get our astronauts safely to Mars and home again. As you now know, it's also the best age-reversal program ever developed. With AstroFit's comprehensive guide to gaining muscle and bone, losing body fat, and improving balance, you can add years to your life. My purpose in developing this program was not simply to inhibit aging but to make whatever years you may enjoy in this life as vibrant and fulfilling as they can be. E-Centric exercise is the cornerstone of this proactive, life-enhancing program.

By the time you spend ninety days on AstroFit, you will become an "experiment of one." You will witness a great transformation as you put on calorie-burning muscle. Yet I'm sure that not only will you look different, but you will *feel* transformed as well. You will undergo both a physical and emotional transformation.

AstroFit is all about change. In three months I want you to achieve your personal short- and long-term goals. I want you to become stronger and more limber. Following the AstroFit nutrition suggestions, you will eat with purpose and pleasure. You will feel younger and more confident and find that you have control of your own destiny. By realizing the potential you find within yourself, you'll be empowered to effectively alter the course of your life.

It will feel great. And you will deserve all the credit.

The formula for your success is straightforward and progressive: Accomplish more than you did the previous day, week, or twelve weeks before. Keep track in your diary of the advances you make, thereby measuring your progress. As I've already mentioned, in order to make progress, it must be measured.

Keep your AstroFit chart with you, and keep taking your measurements. Don't forget to have a complete set of current photographs taken in your bathing suit. Place the before and after shots next to each other, and you'll have all the evidence you need to let you know that you have been successful in your efforts.

But what happens after the first ninety days of following the AstroFit program, exercising regularly, and following the suggested meal plans and recipes to bring about your remarkable transformation? You'll have come a long way, and after three months of this discipline, you will have built a solid foundation for continued success.

Set some new short- and long-term goals for yourself. Start a new twelve-week diary. Make the commitment to integrating AstroFit into your way of life. Transformation is not a one-shot deal; rather, it will be your new reality.

All transformation is subject to challenge from your old ways, and there will be plenty of roadblocks and assorted obstacles. Just like the astronauts, you may require some course corrections. They will help you get back on track as quickly as possible.

The AstroFit program is designed to relieve stress, not cause it. Don't be too hard on yourself if you can't live up to certain daily goals. Nobody's perfect. Missing a planned workout doesn't mean that your program is doomed. Get back to your regular routine as soon as possible. Don't become discouraged or disappointed if you should falter. Refer to your diary often. Bolster your self-esteem with this chronicle of personal achievement. Be proactive. Go public with your success. Engage with the world in a physical way that continues to reinforce the gains you have made.

The AstroFit program will now serve as your personal blueprint for a new way of living. Set goals to become even stronger. Continue planning your workouts with those goals clearly in mind. You'll know you're succeeding if you are doing more repetitions or lifting heavier weights than before and your body recovers faster from a workout.

The clock is ticking, but it can certainly be slowed, even turned back, so you'll look and feel your best. As John Donne said, "Death comes equally to us all, and makes us all equal when it comes." Our choice, then, is how we choose to live. The AstroFit program will make you feel better, look better, and, it is hoped, live longer.

To your good health!

Appendix A: The Best Methods of Measuring Body Fat Percentage

How much you weigh is not a very good indicator of your success on the AstroFit program because your bathroom scale can't distinguish between pounds that come from body fat and those that come from muscle or lean body mass. For example, George, a five-foot, eight-inch man who weighs 175 pounds and has 15 percent body fat, is probably fitter than Richard, a man of the same height who tips the scales at 155 and has 26 percent body fat.

Unfortunately, your scale can never give you this vital bit of information, so you'll have to get it elsewhere. That's where body fat testing comes in.

Many medical centers, as well as some health clubs and doctor's offices, offer body fat measurement tests. You can even purchase a home model that looks—but doesn't act—like a traditional bathroom scale. Just remember that each measuring device has its own . level of imprecision and it's difficult to get a 100 percent accurate reading, so use the results only as a basic guide. Here are the most common body fat tests currently available:

Dual Energy X-Ray Absorptiometry (DEXA)

What the Test Is. DEXA uses two X-ray energies to measure body fat, muscle, and bone mineral density. Many women are already familiar with DEXA because the same technology is used to measure bone density during their test for osteoporosis. The uniqueness of this machine is that it not only reveals your total percentage of body fat but also indicates where the fat is located on your trunk, arms, and legs. When having the scan performed, you lie on a table similar to one used for X rays, while the machine scans your body. When the newer fan beam DEXA is used (the extremely low radiation sweeps over the body in a broad fan fashion), the testing takes five minutes. If the older machine, with its narrower pencil beam, is used, testing can take up to twenty minutes.

Where to Have It Done. Prices range from $50 to $100 and higher. While most hospitals have the machine, many of the diagnosticians using it don't have the correct software to perform body composition measurements. To find where you can have a DEXA body composition test performed, contact your local diagnostic center or hospital.

Advantages
- The test is quick and accurate.
- Radiation exposure is low.
- No special preparation is required.

Disadvantages
- The test is expensive.
- It is not readily available.

The BOD POD

What the Test Is. Developed by Life Measurement, Inc., of Concord, California, this futuristic egg-shaped capsule uses air displacement to measure your total body volume. Stripped to latex shorts and wearing a tightly fitted bathing cap, you sit comfortably in the POD's cabin for a few minutes, breathing normally and refraining from moving. Computerized sensors determine the amount of air displaced by your body, yielding an extremely accurate body fat measurement in a matter of minutes.

Where to Have It Done. Testing costs around $35, with prices ranging from $25 to $100 nationwide. For individual body fat testing, call the company at (800)-4-BODPOD) for the site nearest you.

Advantage
- The test is fast and accurate.

Disadvantages
- The test is expensive.
- It is not widely available.

Underwater Weighing

What the Test Is. The Greek scientist Archimedes stated long ago that when a body is submerged in water, there is a buoyant counterforce that's equal to the weight of water that has been displaced. While Archimedes was certainly correct, underwater weighing is cumbersome. In order to be tested, you wear a bathing suit and weighted belt and then sit or kneel on a chair suspended in a tank of water. After expelling all of the air from your lungs, you dunk your head under the water. Usually at least three measurements are taken. The average figure is then compared to your weight on land, and an equation is applied to figure the percentage of body fat.

Where to Have It Done. The only place to get yourself hydrostatically weighed is at a university exercise physiology or human performance lab. Testing may cost up to $100.

Advantage
- The test is accurate.

Disadvantages
- The test is expensive.
- It is not widely available.

Bioelectrical Impedance (BI)

What the Test Is. In bioelectrical impedance testing, electrodes are attached to your ankles and feet and an imperceptible electric charge is then sent through your body. Since fat is a very poor conductor of electricity, it impedes the current. More resistance means more fat.

For the most accurate BI measurement, I recommend that you not consume any alcoholic beverages for forty-eight hours before the test. Do not exercise twelve hours beforehand, and abstain from eating and drinking for four hours before the test. Also, urinate completely before the test is given. This test consistently overestimates the fat content of lean, muscular people by as much as 2 to 5 percent and underestimates that of obese people by the same margin.

Where to Have It Done. A popular fixture in many health clubs, the machine requires virtually no skill to operate and testing takes less than a minute. Prices vary from nothing to $25. Home monitors are also available. To get a reading, you stand barefoot on metal foot plates (Tanita Body Fat Monitor) or have low-current electricity sent from one hand to the other (Omron Body Fat Analyzer). The prices of these devices, which are sold in department and fitness stores, range from $100 to $400.

Advantages
- The test is accurate, easy to perform, and quick.
- Testing can be done at your convenience at home.

Disadvantage
- The machine has a standard error range.

Skinfold Measurement

What the Test Is. Highly accurate when performed by a well-trained person, this test involves pinching the skin together at three to seven sites on the body. A skinfold caliper—a simple two-armed plastic measurement tool specifically designed for accurate measurement of subcutaneous tissue—is then used to measure the folds.

Where to Have It Done. You can purchase your own calipers (prices range from $25 for basic calipers to $220 for a professional model) to do this test at home. However, the test's accuracy depends on the skill of the person taking the measurements. Inexperience can yield results that vary wildly from one test to another. Have the same person do the test each time.

Advantages
- The calipers are easy to use once the skill has been mastered.
- The test is quick, noninvasive, and affordable.

Disadvantage
- Accuracy relies on the ability of the tester.

Ultrasound

What the Test Is. This test is based on the principles of light absorption. A computerized device that has a scan and probe is placed on the biceps. It emits an infrared light, which passes through both fat and muscle and is reflected back to the probe. Using computerized calculations based on your height, weight, sex, age, frame size, and activity level, your density measurements from the ultrasound are then incorporated into the body fat prediction equation (which is based on the amount of fat in a biceps).

How Do You Measure Up?
BODY FAT RANGES FOR MEN

Optimal: 10 to 15 percent
Average: 18 to 23 percent
Obese: 25 percent or more

BODY FAT RANGES FOR WOMEN

Optimal: 17 to 22 percent
Average: 25 to 29 percent
Obese: 35 percent or more

Note: At any age, the healthy range of body fat is significantly higher for women than for men. This is because women need extra body fat for reproductive function.

Where to Have It Done. Ultrasound testing is widely available in health clubs and hospitals, with fees ranging from nothing to $40. A home testing version (Futrex) is also available. Although this test is fast, convenient, and easy, the results are not very accurate when compared to those of the other instruments.

Advantage
- The test is safe, noninvasive, fast, and affordable.

Disadvantage
- The test is not the most accurate.

Tips For Successful Body Fat Testing

To be sure you're obtaining the most accurate measurements from these devices, here are four important tips:

1. Since measurements can vary among the various devices, choose one method and stick with it for all of your subsequent measurements.
2. Body fat percentages take time to change, so measure yourself *monthly* under similar conditions. The time of day can affect the results, so if, for instance, you start by measuring yourself in the morning, continue to take your measurements in the morning.
3. Refrain from eating or exercising for two hours before being tested.
4. Dehydration can throw the results off, so drink plenty of water before your test.

Index

About the Authors

William J. Evans, Ph.D., a pioneer in the field of age reversal for more than twenty years, has worked as an expert adviser to NASA on nutrition and exercise since 1988, and is the former head of the Nutrition, Physical Fitness, and Rapid Rehabilitation Team of the National Space Biomedical Institution. He lives in Little Rock, Arkansas, with his wife and three children.

Gerald Secor Couzens is the managing editor of *The Johns Hopkins Prostate Bulletin* and a contributing writer for both the *Johns Hopkins Health After 50* newsletter and the Johns Hopkins White Papers medical series. He lives in New York City with his wife and four children.

9 780743 216821

Made in the USA
Monee, IL
22 October 2020

45824662R00194